DISMANTLING
THE TREE OF KNOWLEDGE OF
GOOD AND EVIL WITHIN
SO LOVE CAN THRIVE

RENE LAFAUT, MSc.

DEDICATION

I dedicate this book to all those who struggle navigating relationships.
Those who have compulsive behaviors, and addictions.

ENDORSEMENT

It shows a great amount of wisdom concerning the Christian life that has been learned in the trenches. It shows grace and love rather than a bare legalism.

Bill Reimer, Regent College, Vancouver, BC

Table of Contents

ACKNOWLEDGMENTS

I'd like to acknowledge my family and friends for believing in me,
as I painfully arrived at the content found in this book.

I also want to acknowledge father George Aquaro for his insight into the connections between the seven deadly sins, that helped me so much in my personal development.

Foreword by Rev. Alex Angioli

Many years have passed since I first met Rene Lafaut in the offices of Christian Life Center in downtown Vancouver. Rene was involved in studies toward his PhD in Mathematics at University of British Columbia and had started having some disturbing experiences that interfered with his studies. He came to me as a professional counsellor who he hoped would be of use in sorting out the difficulties he was experiencing.

My memories of that time tend to move toward one issue and that was Rene's steadfast allegiance and insistence on the Lordship of Jesus Christ and his struggle to remain steadfast on this issue. Even after I referred him to a psychiatrist whose anti-faith stance attempted to cause him to abandon his faith, I recall how forthrightly Rene rejected that man's mistaken suggestions. The many challenges to Rene's depth of understanding as a thinker and as a faithful believer would mount going forward to challenges that most people would find petrifying. But this foreword is not an introduction to Rene's spiritual life. He can decide whether to explore that particular topic independently.

As a foreword, I would like to touch on some aspects of Rene's ideas that I believe reach to aspects of the rootedness of Christian life. One of the ways we can understand the Christian life is by way of the story. Now I am not referring to the underlying reality of the story of Jesus himself here, but a secondary yet powerful account of a leader of the church.

Augustine of Hippo (354-430) occupies the position of the most outstanding Christian author, outside the New Testament, whose story of faith and struggles with a variety of heresies marks the beginning and the standard of spiritual story in world history. From the standpoint of the history of literature, the writings of Augustine stand as a foundational source for the literary development of the 'story of one's life'. The paradigm of the struggle between the city of God and that of the world is the key to his personal journey of faith. Augustine's story of the journey from the secular city (Rome) to the city of God (Jerusalem) signals the story of Augustine's own life - his grasp of the fundamentals of the Christian faith and his journey away from heresy.

Rene's searching approach to the spiritual life draws from roots similar to Augustine's, skillfully weaving personal history and challenges to the needs of the individual struggle in the spiritual dynamics. He moves beyond the challenges of moving out of oppression to a possible expansion of spiritual insight. Possibly too detailed in his approach to certain aspects of the struggle between good and evil for some readers, others will find that Rene's examination of the spiritual life sheds a welcome light into dynamics which have become overlaid by the short views of 21st century seekers. Truth needs work, not a 10-second solution.

"Only by focusing on the goal, and focusing on the grace, truths and promises of God will we be able to make it through the messiness of life. Without a goal, or a healthy focus we are more susceptible to the lies of the devil, he will do whatever is in his power to torment us, neutralize us, and draw us away from the straight and narrow path before us." (R. Lafaut, p.24).

Now we do not need to compare ourselves to the genius of Augustine but we do need to take authority for the spiritual direction of our lives, and so we are drawn by the mystery and the contradictions of a free will and a dependent sinfulness; the inspiration of a divine invitation and the dependence of our spiritual destiny on the divine force at work in Jesus Christ himself.

It is a Christian responsibility to know, study and make progress in spiritual maturity from the wisdom of the Orthodox to the post-modern understanding of the faith. No one is exempt from knowledge on one hand, and humble aspiration to humility and comprehension on the other.

Rene's summary of the disciplines needed to confront the spiritual struggle come from a heartfelt personal confrontation with the deceptions of self and the devil and represent a mystical tradition of self-examination and outward responsibility that falls in line with spiritual thinkers through the ages.

Truth is the standard, so readers of this book are invited to face their own truth, and to make progress under the guidance of God's Spirit.

Rev. Alex Angioli

Missionary of the Anglican Church AMIC

MTS, DipMin, STM, MA Counselling Psychology

1 Introduction

This book was written in response to questions I had accumulated over the years, as I struggled with getting rid of "sin strongholds" (those things that go against self-love, people-love, and God-love), that I was powerless to change all by myself. I confessed my struggles to spiritual directors, priests, and those I trusted with my baggage, over many years. But I felt none of them had the necessary experience, or had lived with as hard a heart or as confused a mind like I had, to fully deal with my issues; they had never walked in my shoes. Yet, I was open to the wisdom that came my way and helped me to navigate life until the contents of this book were slowly revealed and successfully administered to me in prayer.

Ultimately, I ended up embracing God, my Bible, and input from the body of Christ[1], and I decided to let them speak to me. I did not have immediate revelations that answered all my questions all at once, but I began to journey with God. And God used uncomfortable circumstances and awkward moments I had with people, to show me what was in my heart, so that we could work on cleaning up my life from the inside out.

The Gospel's invitation to its hearers is to repent and believe in Jesus. However, the word "repent" is often misunderstood, both by those outside and inside the church, because of so much hypocrisy and powerlessness to make it real. The "how-to" part of repentance is not well understood, and very confusing to many people who struggle with sin strongholds and experience guilt, shame, powerlessness, and condemnation from others.

Personally, I began to discover that my vocabulary, understanding, and practice of basic Christian tenets was weak, and that led to me searching for revelations on how to repent from my strongholds of sin; and how to change my negative, unloving attitudes to become a more positive person—with Jesus' gracious help, promises, and truth found in Scripture. I started to learn how to process my emotional baggage within and how to navigate my conflicts with others in a more healthy manner. The "how-to" part was not immediately obvious to me for the longest time even though I believed I was a Christian who had gone through many serious trials without losing my faith.

Having said this, many people go to church thinking everything is right in their souls: they have supposedly arrived, they are the correct package, or they keep all the rules (and they think that they belong for such reasons). But none of us are the complete package; only Jesus is. The fact is, we sin—sometimes grossly and sometimes repeatedly. If we are honest, we realize that even

---

[1] Cf. Chapter fourteen for those authors whose books helped to point me in healthy directions so I could eventually enter more deeply into the healing process that Jesus was leading me through.

with cleaning up the outside, there are often many unresolved issues or sinful habits that we likely don't have the desire, commitment, energy or know-how to overcome. We often focus only on one or two issues in our lifetime because we don't know how to start cleaning up even a little of the stuff in our hearts that we feel guilty about. We don't understand what is happening in our hearts that causes us to sin habitually.

I am learning to conquer many of the sin strongholds in my life, through Jesus' promises, teachings, commands, authority, power (grace), truths, and presence. And I want to share how I am experiencing this process with you. Having said this, I am a sinner and I ask for grace when receiving communion; I don't earn it. Confessing sin and working on repentance is more important to God than preparing to receive communion by abstaining from all visible sins just prior to communion. A thorough cleaning job is better than cosmetic changes; if I can repent from serious sin, I should do so, to restore myself to a state of grace.

The invitation from God that I accepted, to change for spiritual and relational health reasons, isn't based on deep mysteries, or complex doctrines, but on the basic teachings of Jesus Christ. But this Good News was forgotten by me soon after conversion, discounted as "too easy to be true," and later jettisoned as only being important for "baby-Christians." The reason I didn't make progress for a long time and didn't grow into maturity as a Christian is because I thought I knew better and had moved onto greener pastures. However, real change comes slowly and only comes to those who don't give up, to those who do search for how to care for and love people, and to those that don't discount or despise the simplicity of the Gospels.

There is a lot of theology in this book that I use to support my take on how I've learned to repent. It should not be looked at as a system, or set of laws that need to be conformed to for there to be freedom. Freedom only comes from abiding in Jesus and He lets us know, when we are listening, what needs to be believed and practiced. No finite set of rules, principles, or codes is enough to solve all our problems—and this applies to this book. Rules create pressure not freedom; but healthy relationships do create freedom. So, if God speaks to you in some context through this book, embrace it when it happens, but the focus should always be on what Jesus is showing you.

As with all books that talk about the possibility of change, there is a caution with this one. When I have been set free by a truth and grace, in an area that may have plagued me for decades, my impulse has often been to carry the truth to an extreme. I forget about grace, I get proud, and I start to judge and hurt people because of my twisted slant on things. Unfortunately, church history has witnessed many people in authority trying to muzzle truths that seem dangerous and threatening to them or the status quo. Whatever the place of authority in the church is, and they do have a place, if one can't embrace truth, one embraces fear. When I encounter a new truth I usually don't grasp all of its aspects immediately. I need to wrestle with it until I understand its limitations, and its freeing power through grace. I need the freedom to make mistakes and that means sometimes taking things too far. Without this freedom to make mistakes I wouldn't learn and grow in the freedom to love or mature like I have.

The Gospel of John says Jesus is full of grace and truth. I have learned that I need Jesus and the grace and truth He offers, if I want my sin strongholds to lose their power and their structures to be dismantled.

The sin strongholds I speak about in this book erected an ugly superstructure in my heart for a very long time, and can fittingly be called "the tree of knowledge of good and evil" within. And this structure needed to be replaced with love. I have learned some tools to do just that in this book.

"The tree of knowledge of good and evil" is a structure made from commitments to beliefs and expectations based on lies, sin, guilt, and fears rooted in wounds from broken relationships that negatively impact our relational lives.

The three major categories of sin: "unhealthily seeking power", "sex", and "money" characterize "the tree of knowledge of good and evil"; with its building blocks: the trunk: "foolishness, fear and pride," and its two major branches: "abandoning love, compulsive-laziness, compulsive-indulging" and "coveting, judging, selfishness" respectively. These are commonly revealed to us through broken relationships, business dealings, wars, history, the news, TV, radio, internet, movies, magazines, or read about in books. In rejecting God, we seek power to carry out our plans to survive, and to make a name for ourselves just like those who built the Tower of Babel, as is recorded in the book of Genesis. Just as many people in the church are growing this hideous tree within themselves, as those outside of the church. We are all fallen.

 "The tree of knowledge of good and evil" within us, consists of a dark energy stretching and giving life to those detestable building blocks and branches of bad fruit. It needs to be dismantled for love to thrive.

Here is an overview of this book:

- Chapter 1 is the introduction.

- In chapter 2, I talk about the power of the "sin nature" vs. "the tree of knowledge of good and evil" within me, and how they differ on their impact in my life. Understanding this helps me to choose my battles wisely.

- In chapter 3, I give a description of the methodology (summed up in the Twelve-Principles) God gave me so I could enter a deeper transforming friendship with Him, like He promised me a long time ago. This chapter shows what I learned to expect from God, and what energy and humility is needed for real change.

- In chapter 4, I start to describe how I've learned to dismantle "the tree of knowledge of good and evil" within me. I give key Scriptures that are used to drive the methodology and some definitions of Christian jargon that make transformation possible in this life; without them little but cosmetic change is possible. In the next five chapters, I attempt to show the connections between the different parts belonging to "the tree of knowledge of good and evil," to help us pray through them more thoroughly and help to dismantle them in the varying contexts of our lives.

- In chapter 5, I expand my discussion on the process of transformation, by talking about broken relationships and our search for peace in the wrong places—which is where "the tree of knowledge of good and evil" deceptively comes from.

- In chapter 6, I explain how to heal fear and its related vices, which are a part of "the tree of knowledge of good and evil." I talk about healing self-pity, worry, pressure, cowardice, and conceit which are all ingredients that allow the tree to grow wildly.

- In chapter 7, I explain how to kill the stronghold of pride from the tree, and grow humility instead. Deeply renewing the mind with healthy, strategic truths and thinking, is key to stopping the tree's growth. Arrogance, pressure, and using force are also related ingredients that allow this tree to grow wildly.

- In chapter 8, I explain how I stop using people, and prune the related vices of compulsive-laziness and compulsive-indulging from "the tree of knowledge of good and evil" and how I grow healthy habits instead.

- In chapter 9, I explain how I give up my coveting, envious and jealous ways, and prune the related vices of judging, anger, addiction, moral policing, greed, and selfishness from the "tree of knowledge of good and evil," and how to grow kindness and generosity instead.

- In chapter 10, I summarize what was discussed in the previous chapters and provide troubleshooting tips if you get stuck.

- Chapter 11, I give six successful personal examples of how to work and pray so certain parts of "the tree of knowledge of good and evil" can be dismantled within you.

- Chapter 12, I present an alternative tree to replace "the tree of knowledge of good and evil" whose source is God and is accessed through a humble faith relationship.

- Chapter 13 outlines my conclusion.

There are many graphic and coarse examples of sin strongholds in this book. They are brutal, ugly, selfish, proud, arrogant, hostile, mean, hurtful, and often angry—and, they are mine. They sprout from unhealthy beliefs that grew their way into my subconscious, as I foolishly tried to suppress emotional baggage and not process any of it in a healthy manner.

Whenever I believed a devil's lie about myself and the people I knew, a false thought pattern was formed and over the years these developed into strongholds. As these were reinforced and other negative thought patterns added to it resulted in a tangled mess that had little basis in reality, functioned mainly from my subconscious mind and made a huge mess in my interior and relational life. I ended up stuffing away the bad energy that came from inside of me, and I kept believing the devil's lies for years. I didn't know how to wash away what was inside of me, even though I wanted to be clean. I did not know how to get healed, but I really wanted the healing. I did not like my lack of love and I did not know what to do about it until God gave me the answers found in this book. Lies usually sound good to us when we believe them, but the consequences of doing so are often horrible. Lies always have catches.

Words of advice:

1. Don't isolate yourself: I did not find any healing when I isolated myself and put my own needs selfishly before others. The parable of the Good Samaritan illustrates this well: it has a priest who cares more about his spiritual state than a wounded person on the side of the road. When I care more about "not sinning" than loving the people in my life, then I won't grow in God's grace. The way to healing is to seek to love, and that means putting people before concepts and other idols. Seeking to love—not waiting until I'm healthy enough, or until it is easier to love—is the path to growing in love. I see difficulties and obstacles as my classroom in this process of learning to love.

2. Acknowledge you are God's instrument: I don't produce good fruit, but I bear it—to use the True Vine allegory from John 15. All of the virtues (goodness, love, compassion, mercy, and grace) that come out of me are a result of the Holy Spirit. He performs His work through me. I am an instrument God uses. A long time ago, God told me that He was digging tunnels of love within me. When I love, the Holy Spirit lives in me and uses me as His instrument of love. God gets the glory.

   > I have been crucified with Christ and I no longer live, but Christ lives in me. The life I now live in the body, I live by faith in the Son of God, who loved me and gave himself for me.[2]

---

[2] Galatians 2:20

Admitting that I am God's instrument is what honest pride acknowledges. I concede that God is the Author, Mastermind, Life Giver, and Peace Giver that is responsible for whatever good comes out of me. When Paul says, "We no longer live," he means we no longer live according to the flesh or "sin nature" but we are now dedicated to the Holy Spirit.

3. Keep your attention on God: Focusing primarily on Jesus' presence and grace, and secondly on little "t" truths that are God's wisdom spoken into the situation at hand. This will bring stability in navigating life's obstacles to love, because they keep me from using anger and self-pity for selfish reasons.

4. Don't just go through the motions: I no longer assume that doing things that require effort will always become easy through prayers, or that by coasting through life I can do God's will. Going by what feels good is never a good idea when it comes to living a healthy life. Practicing self-control, doing acts of love, and working in a useful manner is the path to life. If I do abandon effort, initiative and caring, and instead coast through life seeking pleasure, then I negate the useful strategies found in this book. And "the tree of knowledge of good and evil" will not die, and the "flesh" or "sin nature" will help to strengthen this tree's domination over our relationships.

All sins that attempt to get us what we desire end up hurting others: exploitation, greed, compulsive-laziness, selfishness, pride, judging, compulsive-indulging, angry pressure, force, hatred, and meanness directed at others and ourselves to better our positions in life, or acquire material things, or spiritual things we covet. It all ends up hurting us immediately and stays with us on into the future, if not processed healthily. The strategies outlined in this book helped me learn to love myself, others, and God more deeply. We can't love God if we don't love others and ourselves. When I pray, like I suggest in this book, I have often got in touch with and felt the powerful rawness and intense sensitivity of the wound within me. And I eventually realized that I needed to learn how to love myself to help the raw wound be healed. If I don't love myself, God's love can't get through to me, or as deeply as I need Him too.

Asking God to heal the sin within me, confessing the sin I commit against myself and others, repenting in prayer, renewing my mind and attitudes towards myself and others, gently submitting to God daily and resisting the devil—all help to bring inner and relational healing to me.

All sin strongholds are immature, self-centered, and self-pitying. The way for me to progress has been to uproot my bad attitudes—by giving up the lies and immature beliefs I had incorporated into my whole life: my thinking, my beliefs, my personality, my character, my actions, and my internal structures. I couldn't take giant leaps to maturity overnight. I realized that each lesson needed to be fully explored, understood, put into practice.

"God comforts me, consoles me, refreshes me but He does not want me to become stuck with

Him forever changing my diapers, so He wisely puts challenges or things that bring discomfort in my path to urge me forward to growth so my path doesn't become stagnant."[3]

I found that I must fully master each lesson in order for progress to be made, so that what St. Paul said could eventually come true in my life:

> When I was a child, I talked like a child, I thought like a child, I reasoned like a child. When I became a man, I put the ways of childhood behind me.[4]

Sometimes we can have very valid concerns but the methodology to stand up for them or to carry them out can be very unhealthy. The mode in which we attempt to carry out good causes can either be childish or mature. It can be done or demanded crudely, meanly, angrily, in self-pity; this all needs to be jettisoned. Valid concerns still need to be embraced, but with gentleness, respect, kindness, honor, peace, and acceptance; we can't demand things to always go our way. Instead we submit in kindness, letting the truth speak up for itself.

Even when we have a good cause we can be mean and judgmental, and proudly, intolerantly developing and carrying out our cause. This needs to be repented from.

You might notice, in starting to read this book, that you feel more judgmental in some ways. If this is the case, then the book is triggering what has only been hidden from you in your heart and mind up until now. As one perseveres in applying the principles found in this book, what is in you that gets triggered will eventually be dismantled, with Jesus' grace and truth. And you will become more tolerant, compassionate, caring, and loving towards the people in your life. So don't give up reading and applying this book to your life.

The book of James, in chapter 3, says (and I paraphrase): "where the tongue goes, the body follows suit." I'm pained at how true this has been in my life when I speak negatively. When I seek to control situations or people I use my words. With my speech, I judge what is pleasurable and I hurt people. "The tree of knowledge of good and evil" within me is heavily influenced by how I use my tongue: lies spring from my tongue, lies caused this tree to grow stronger and more twisted over time, and lies helped me hurt others. My tongue speaks from the abundance of what is stored in my heart either for good or for evil. What is stored in my heart are my beliefs, loyalties, desires, and commitments; and I often end up believing what I carelessly speak.

It is fitting then, that through prayer (the tongue) and with God's help, this unhealthy "tree of knowledge of good and evil" within me can be dismantled. This is usually a gradual process, and it is a good idea to say the prayers we learn to craft in this book repeatedly, going deeper until

---

[3] This thought comes from my friend Mark Munn.
[4] 1 Corinthians 13:11

the strongholds are completely dismantled and uprooted. Also, learning to give thanks to God for the practical progress, forgiveness, and healing that come our way helps to brighten our attitudes and lessen the unwanted burdens. It's all about freedom to love.

This book is about inner healing. Sin in the Bible is defined as spiritual sickness. When we are healed from the sin within us (think sin strongholds), then we become healthy again and freedom results in that area.

If you need to repent, then the approach found in this book is useful, but the enemy is not always the "sin nature" or "the tree of knowledge of good and evil." In some cases, demonization and delusional types of mental illnesses may need to be addressed as possible diagnoses and healed with other medicines, especially when repenting does not work in certain contexts of one's life.

Asked by a reader if I am growing in compassion, love, and caring for people as I apply the steps and principles found in my book, I responded to her very assuredly: "Yes". The book requires work from the reader for it to be of benefit. One need not outright memorize the steps found in the third chapter (as we often put them in practice daily without even thinking about them). I think that just reading through the book to see where it goes is a helpful first step and to not get bogged down in the details at first. Once one sees where the book goes then one can pray through the Sin-Conduit Structures found in one's personal "tree of knowledge of good and evil" like I show in the book. This has been life changing for me, and I believe it can be life-changing for the reader too.

There is a pain in processing and dismantling the tree within each of us. It's facing the negative energy and bad commitments from the past that got to be strongholds in our lives. This can form a dread and a reluctance to do the work necessary to find freedom to love God and neighbors like oneself. Fighting through this takes grace and the realization that one won't get free otherwise.

2 The Power Of My Sin Nature Vs. The Tree Of Knowledge Of Good And Evil Within

"The tree of knowledge of good and evil" is not the same as the "sin nature." Why is it that one person has no addictions, while another can't stop eating or getting drunk? Why is it that one person has spiritual pride, whereas another is humble about spiritual things? Why is it that one person gets jealous so easily, while another person is more altruistic? Is one person's "sin nature" better than another person's "sin nature"? No, there is a level playing field. But we can allow our "sin nature," together with our choices and folly, to grow "the tree of knowledge of good and evil" in us; a structure of death and bad fruit (hatred, malice, addictions and negativity) that tries to push everyone away from us.

Yes, the "sin nature" can make us judge, worry, be proud, be jealous, be greedy, focus on selfish love, overeat, and be lazy. But these only become strongholds when they become compulsive, and when they do, they form a part of the structure within that is called "the tree of knowledge of good and evil." And this tree is merciless.

If the tree of knowledge of good and evil is the very first introduction to mankind about knowing good from evil, then the temptation in the garden of Eden seems unfair and confusing. It must have been a set-up for failure. If Adam and Eve had no knowledge of good and evil before they ate from the tree of knowledge of good and evil, then who could blame them? If we don't understand the nature and purpose of this tree then we will not be able to understand how it affects each of us. Understanding the nature of this tree is crucial to weakening its power and influence over each of us and mankind.

The tree of knowledge of good and evil did not introduce the ideas of good and evil to mankind. The devil promised Adam and Eve an understanding of good and evil but withheld from them that they would end up using evil in trying to get good things. The tree enticed Adam and Eve with what looked like an easier way to get things. And the human family still buys into this trap daily.

Yes, Adam and Eve partially knew good and evil in the sense that God did before the temptation in the garden of Eden. This tree is really a tree of sin because it came in between humankind and God. It is an unhealthy tree. It promises that good will come by doing evil; hence this is its nature. It separated Adam and Eve, and us their fallen descendants, from complete sober dependence on God to do good and to know right from wrong.

Instead, it set up a paradigm of thought where foolishness, fear, and pride became the means to getting good things. Sin is using evil means to getting the desired good. The desired good is never as good as is promised when we get it in an under-handed way. We are often full of guilt, self-loathing, anger, and emptiness after we buy into the devil's lie – the lie that the tree of knowledge of good and evil will give us what we want and we end up doing what it asks.

The tree of knowledge of good and evil is a shortcut to getting what we think we want. It needs to be dismantled and removed from within each of us. To do this we need knowledge of what this tree looks like and how it functions within us. In this book I give a language, understanding, and tools that can be used to dismantle this tree within each of us. Each person has their own tree, but a God-given strategy can help dismantle the tree so love can thrive. We need Jesus along with His grace and truth for this to work.

In this chapter, I develop a rationale for how "the tree of knowledge of good and evil" develops within us, and is acted on by the "sin nature"; fear and pride in the context of relational conflicts, challenges, and foolishness. The diagram[5] below shows two-continuums of behavior where we can find ourselves. In the center is the place of humility, where there is awareness of our self-preservation and connectedness to our altruism; these two natures are healthy God-given qualities.

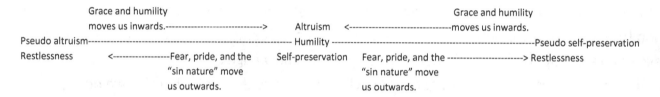

But within us is a dark energy, force, or pull known as the "sin nature" or the "flesh" that tries to pull us away from humility (spiritual healthiness) through fear (of having to love in sacrificial ways), and pride. We are driven towards extremes on both sides: pseudo self-preservation (coveting, jealousy, and selfishness) on the right, and pseudo altruism (lust or selfish-love) on the left (pseudo meaning "not genuine"). I have found that when I grow in humility I move along either continuum towards the center, but even when I am near the center I will feel my self-preservation and altruism being pulled and harassed by the "sin nature." One can get self-preservation confused with selfishness when one doesn't understand the pull of the "sin nature." When I don't jump the gun and patiently wait, then I see the difference. The more one moves away from the center the more one acts out of lies that inspire fear and pride.

The sense of self-preservation within us is strong, and we need to acknowledge it as a gift from God. The pull to the right by the "sin nature", through fear and pride is strong too, and should not be ignored. To annihilate the "sin nature" is an impossibility in this life. Yes, I can kill the strongholds of fear and pride, but I can't kill the "sin nature" within me. God grants me grace,

---

[5] I am grateful to my friend Rafael for a discussion that inspires this diagram

truth, and strategies to say, "I accept you, but I don't need you right now," [6] directly to the "sin nature." When these attitudes rear their ugly heads (usually through angry pressure mixed with self-pity and possibly ugly demands), I pray: "I give it up, with your help Jesus, through faith"; so I can say yes to Jesus' peace (known as the Holy Spirit); and I ask Him to overcome my sin instead. [7] But I will always feel the pull to the extreme right in this life.

My sense of altruism is strong too, and I need to acknowledge it as a gift from God, not as a badge of honor that gets me God's favor. The "sin nature" tries to draw me to the left: congratulating me on noble acts; trying to motivate me with fears of rejection and losses of honor; trying to move me with pride and conceit; and pushing me towards a reputation of goodness that is actually full of selfish-love, empty love, and self-righteousness. The fear is one of not being accepted, welcomed, loved, and cared for. My conceit in action (also known as "the ego" going bad) actually steals genuine honor and real love directed towards me, and I need to say, "I accept you, but I don't need you right now" to it. When this dark energy within rears its ugly head, then I pray, "I give it up, with your help Jesus, through faith"; so I can say, yes to Jesus' peace (known as the Holy Spirit), and ask I Him to overcome my sin. It's important to note, that in saying, "no" to the "sin nature" I give it a firmer place in my life to tempt me that it doesn't deserve.

"It is in dying that we are born again," comes from a prayer inspired by St. Francis of Assisi's life, and it is often used in conjunction with St. Paul's statement: "For me to live is Christ, to die is gain,"[8] These might seem to justify the idea that we can kill the "sin nature" but in fact this is impossible. We incorrectly put pressure on ourselves to do this through anger and self-hatred so we can somehow love people more deeply, but this is a horrible trap. We can't crucify ourselves or our "flesh", and we can't kill the "sin nature"; but we can kill the strongholds mentioned in this book with Jesus' help. When St. Paul used the word "die" he was referring to physical death and being united with Jesus in heaven. We can't add anything to Jesus or what He has done to be any better.

When I saw that all people have a "sin nature within, that the Bible calls the "flesh,"[9] then I began to realize that we are all basically the same. There is no need to feel superior to others, to judge others, or to condemn others—and when I do, then I have spiritual pride. No matter how far I walk spiritually in this life, the "flesh" is still with me; any healthy righteousness within me always comes from God. I have nothing to boast about (not even about God's Spirit within me) because I am not better than anyone else.

---

[6] Insight from my friend Suda.
[7] Cf. Romans 8:2,13
[8] Philippians 1:21
[9] Cf. Romans 7:14-20

Pseudo altruism is basically selfish-love—also known as lust. This is illustrated on the left side of the "tree of knowledge of good and evil" below (see diagram). Pseudo self-preservation is basically coveting, jealousy, and selfishness and is illustrated on the right side of the "tree of knowledge of good and evil." Lies inspire fears; and pride together with the "sin nature" try to push me to these two extreme and incomplete perversions of healthy humility.

The power of the "sin nature" works to establish the strongholds of fear, pride, coveting, jealousy, judging, selfishness, using people, compulsive-indulging, compulsive-laziness and the sins that come from them. These strongholds can be dismantled in my life, but the "sin nature" can't be dismantled. The glue that holds this tree-structure together are the lies we believe about the nature of God, people, and ourselves—relationally, and in the context of conflicts, trauma, attacks, and challenges. Lies trigger broken relationships, that trigger fear and guilt, and these work together with the strongholds, and make the "tree of knowledge of good and evil." It is a powerful structure that has sought to dominate humanity since the Garden of Eden.

It is clear that if we have pride, saying we are the center of the universe, then we will seek to use people and things. This is called abandoning love, and that leads to compulsive-laziness (not wanting to love) and compulsive-indulging (seeking pleasure in unhealthy ways to fill the void).

If we have pride, then jealousy results too because we will covet what others have (in a selfish way) and judge others because we think we are better.

These sins of pride, using people, compulsive-indulging, compulsive-laziness, jealousy, judging, and selfishness are not just sins that happen and get relegated to the past. If we let them, they form a bad energy structure of misguided beliefs, commitments, and loyalties in our hearts that leads to a lack of character. This structure grows as we let our foolish loyalties rule, and the only way to change this is to dismantle it. The way I have experienced this structure is like the diagram below:

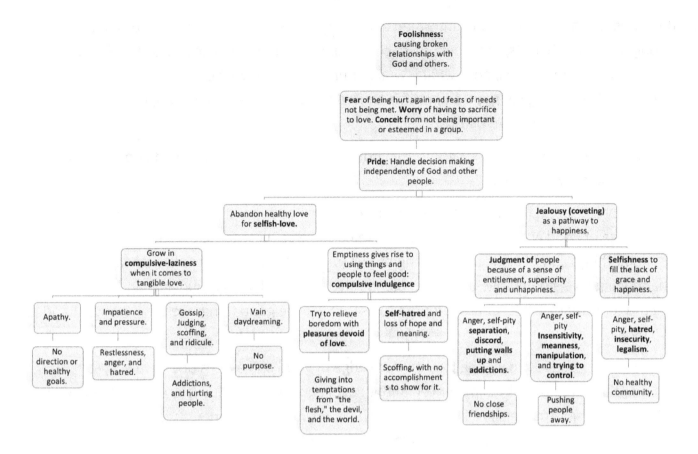

My structure has both similarities and differences to a Tree Diagram put forth by father George Aquaro on his *Orthodoxy and Recovery* blog.[10] Both structures capture truths in their own contexts. His diagram's context is "The state of a man without God"; my diagram's context is about "A broken (imperfect) relationship with God and people" when conflict or trauma enters the scene. His diagram inspired mine and came at the right time.

This tree is a negative energy structure that is held together by hurts, fears, false beliefs and commitments to lies that results in sinful behavior. The very bottom row of the tree contains some of the more visible fruits of indulging in the nature of the tree (many harsher ones can be added). Obviously, this tree does not list all of the sins mentioned in the Bible, but it will do for our discussions. I will show the prescriptions God gave me on how to dismantle this tree within me, and how to replace it with practical life-giving wisdom, with the helping presence of the Holy Spirit.

The "tree of knowledge of good and evil" is an invitation to decide what is good and bad, while ignoring the God who sees everything. We do this when we cut out the cause and effects found in the spiritual realm that God wants us to be informed of, so we can make healthy and wise

---

[10] Inspiration granted from the Mission Statement found in the blog:
http://orthodoxyandrecovery.blogspot.com/

decisions. We aren't always well informed about the physical realm either. There is nothing wrong with our intellects, but when we decide to limit what we can know to space, time, matter, and energy—and ignore what is real but unseen—then we become foolish. The scope of the "tree of knowledge of good and evil" is limited to what we can see through the natural world and our fallen human nature.

The following is how I think the "good" functions in "the tree of knowledge of good and evil" as found in the book of Genesis:

1. Satan promised that Adam and Eve would experience both good and evil through "the tree of knowledge of good and evil." What he didn't tell them was they would end up using the evil to get good things. Sin is taking a good thing by evil (unhealthy) means. Evils like cowardice, pride, abandoning love, compulsive-indulging, compulsive-laziness, jealousy, judging, and selfishness are the tools that we use, or are tempted to use, to get the good things we think we want and to avoid pain.

2. Often, the good found in "the tree of knowledge of good and evil" is one of raising (or idolizing) pleasure (usually experienced in the flesh) and happiness (usually experienced in the mind), above spiritual considerations (what is holy, healthy, and proper, as far as God's design is concerned, when it comes to how we relate to God and each other).

3. The good behavior aimed for in this devilish tree is not rooted in real tangible rightness or spiritually healthy behaviors, as seen in God's nature. It may often look like humility but its source tries to exult in human effort, will, goodness, intellect, and pedigree above God's grace; it is devoid of dependence on God. It is not wise to search this out in people and judge them for it. Jesus is clear: judge and condemn not; leave judgments to God.

4. Pride in the world is often used to measure things as being either "better than" or "worse than", instead of looking at parts of reality as either healthy or unhealthy.

I think that Satan sold the idea to Eve that the "tree of knowledge of good and evil" would get her and Adam to be as "special" as God. He wanted them to think God was holding out on them. The reason I think this is because the "tree of knowledge of good and evil" was the source of a dark kind of thinking where:

> Good =
>
> I'm more special because... or
>
> Mine is more special because... or
>
> You are less special because...

And where:

Evil =

I'm less special because… or

Mine is less special because… or

You are more special because…

This kind of knowledge is a shallow and hurtful paradigm of thought, rooted in disobedience, restlessness, anger, hatred, inferiority, fear and pride. And they bear the rest of the vices that all destroy wholesome, healthy community and peaceful relationships. This kind of knowledge slowly defaces the image of God within us (except for the grace of God in our lives). And in so doing this knowledge helps us to hate, kill, and relish revenge; "eye for an eye and tooth for a tooth" actions against everyone who crosses our paths, eventually seeking the death of all. It is devoid of love, joy, peace, humility, warmth, kindness, hope, gentleness, valuing people, caring, altruism, and being a living sacrifice in the healthiest sense possible.

I have wrongly relied on the "sin nature" to try and save me from things that are uncomfortable in my life; using self-pity and anger to change my interior life, my circumstances, and my relationships. I only end up with guilt, meanness, restlessness, more anger and more self-pity linked to demands for my way to come through in the end—limited only by the presence of grace and mercy given by God.

The seed, structure, and fruit of the "tree of knowledge of good and evil" has infected all humanity: Adam, Eve and us, their fallen descendants. The tree's infecting power is in the lies spoken to us that we too quickly and easily embrace because they promise us many things: instant peace, alleviation of fears, and the lie that God's promises, provisions, and ways through darkness are not trustworthy. The devil promised independence, but made us slaves to sin; only Jesus can free us from this tangled mess through the Good News found in the New Testament (NT).

In this book we will focus on what are called Sin-Conduit Structures that together form "the tree of knowledge of good and evil" within. An example of such a structure is the one traced out below.

One will learn how to confess and repent from these connected sins, attitudes, commitments and habits, with the help of God, and in the process dismantle them, so love can thrive. The dark-arrowed line goes upward because that is the order of how to process the structure and find freedom. The hidden power of each sin stronghold reaches from the roots to the branches of the tree like gravity or suction.

The Sin-Conduit structure below has the shorthand notation (right to left): "Foolishness=> Fear=> Pride=> Coveting and Jealousy=> Judging=> Meanness & Intolerance" in this instance, and fleshed out, can look something like this, with the Sin- Anatomy Table beneath it:

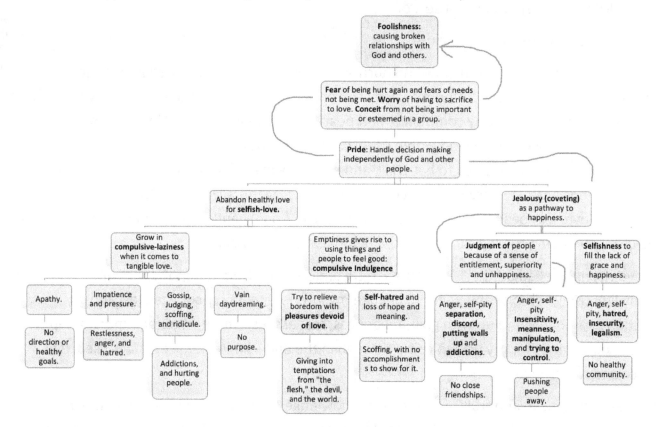

Meanness & Intolerance towards others	Judging	Coveting & Jealousy	Pride	Fear	Foolishness
	<=	<=	<=	<=	<= Cause and Effect
I want my will done (and I choose to do it meanly) instead of aiming for God's will to be done through me: i.e. "that I obey the Golden Rule".	Subconsciously or consciously I demanded: "An eye for an eye, and a tooth for a tooth" treatment towards those in my way... And I actually wanted karma visited on these people instead of grace.	I wanted to get my desires fulfilled ASAP demanding that others cooperate with me so I can get my way.	I see myself as the center of the universe. So my desires are more important than other people's.	I might have to get my hands dirty and love people other than myself. Believing the lie: "Loving people is too hard and unimportant".	People matter only insofar as they help me out with my chosen causes. I am committed to feeling as little pain as possible.
When I treated so and so disrespectfully...					
Confession & Repenting in Faith =>	=>	=>	=>	=>	

I have made many such Sin-Anatomy Tables, confessed and repented from the sins listed within them, and routed strongholds one after another with Jesus' help. I have included some of these tables as they are very helpful in aiming prayers and thoroughly covering all bases. I can't include them all for two reasons:

1. My dirty laundry involves many other people who I don't want to hurt or wound.

2. This book can only be so long.

Most of the prayers said in this book are very general, but keep in mind that I have persons or people in mind when praying them. So when you pray some of these prayers, or construct your own ones be as specific as possible as it will help going deeper with more healing coming your way.

All Sin-Conduit Structures are dark, thirsty, compulsive energies seeking relief, stretching from the root to the branches of "the tree of knowledge of good and evil." It is more like a vacuum, than a supply. It is more like a black hole than a warm sun. These dark energy streams inside me are only concerned about getting and taking things that I think will make me happy (the supposed good). This dark energy doesn't respect people or their boundaries. I need to say to this energy within me, "I accept you but I don't need you"; I need to commit myself to the Holy

Spirit to have victory in each episode where this energy manifests. This dark energy is my "sin nature" and used by "the tree of knowledge of good and evil" within. Sin is about taking and using. Love is about giving and receiving.

It only takes a small situation and sin to start growing "the tree of knowledge of good and evil" within and its growth is not stagnant; it will grow as the years pass if left undealt with. The longer it's left the more gross it gets.

3 The Methodology

Having a vocabulary to describe unwholesome inner emotions, attitudes, and energy is very important in being able to diagnose, to pray more strategically for, and to destroy the sin-strongholds of "the tree of knowledge of good and evil." I have developed such a vocabulary in this book. I know that I have often had *really* bad energy within me, and this vocabulary has helped me to process and deal with it in healthy ways.

There have been repeated times when my energy has been so bad, with me not knowing where it came from. To deal with it I had to pray and ask the Holy Spirit to heal my mind. This was a measure that got me sane enough to get by, but I had to continue to persevere: until I was completely connected to the energy, until I was able to see the lies and pride I held onto, and until I was able to be set free by Jesus' truth and grace.

To annihilate all the "flesh" or to kill the pull towards sin completely—in this life—is not possible. I can though, with Jesus' help, destroy the strongholds of bad attitudes within me, because these are different from the "flesh." But I will always have the "flesh" to deal with in this life. It's natural to experience the "flesh" to some degree when confronted with things in life I do not expect, or when others make requests I have not counted on. Trying to kill the "flesh" is not wise—it is very unhealthy, and comes from a perfectionist mindset which should not be worshipped. It is unhealthy to want to be too righteous. When I expect too much from myself I will expect too much from others and make their lives as miserable as mine.

Canonized saints never considered themselves perfect spiritually in this life. They are often clear thinkers in certain areas of spirituality that the hierarchy and certain segments of the church esteemed. They were very developed in serving others, but not so in all other aspects of life. These saints are special but no more than anyone else. Aiming to serve others like these people did is wise. But we need balance. I thought I was advanced spiritually until horrible attitudes were triggered within me that affected my relationships at home and at work. I struggled with a *big* stronghold of pride, and the tools in this book together with my relationship with God helped dismantle much of it. But I don't expect to kill the "flesh" outright in this life. When I pretend the sinful nature does not exist, it comes back to bite me.

When calamity, chaos, or trauma occur, we all have different reactions. Some of our reactions go really deep, while others are shallow. Some of us feel numb or uncomfortable, while others feel deeply for those involved. Some have waves of sadness, while others feel seething anger. Whatever the reaction in any particular person, unconditional love respects the person and doesn't judge or condemn their reaction.

A long time ago I was made aware of this promise:

> God grants His grace to the humble,
> but opposes the proud.[11]

It is found in both the Old Testament (OT) and NT. By itself, if I do not know my own pride, and what healthy humility looks like, then this promise won't bear any good fruit in my life. But if I know what pride looks like inside of me and what true humility is, then I will have a chance to receive God's grace through his empowering presence. I went through years of not knowing my own pride, and the little I saw I did not know how to humble. I ended up stuffing any knowledge of it away. But when I started to seriously pray for humility and to search for wisdom that could destroy the stronghold of pride, then God started to give me revelations, and I started to see victories in my battles against my pride.

Law vs. Grace

The commandments of Jesus and their relationship to the OT law play a huge role in having victory in the battles against the strongholds of pride and related vices and attitudes. The OT law was a "minimum standard"[12] of behavior between one another, and between humankind and God. The commands of Jesus are higher than the OT Law and are altruistic in nature; submitting to Jesus' commands by grace will inevitably help us to fulfill the OT law. The OT law is very passive and negative in nature compared to the teachings and commands from Jesus found in the NT scriptures. Focusing on the high goal of love, "to do to others what we would want done to us," is key to victory. Too often the "thou shalt not" commands found in the OT are reacted to with, "What is in it for us?" or with rebellion and the desire to do the opposite.

When Jesus says that the Ten Commandments still stand (cf. Matthew 5:17) He is not saying we are under *law* (we are under grace); He is saying that these commandments are still to be used to point out sin. We don't trust in the Ten Commandments to somehow keep them. No, we aim higher than these commandments, like the teachings of Jesus in the Sermon on the Mount outline. In aiming higher, the minimum OT standard will be fulfilled through supernatural love, and prompted through caring and grace poured out through faith in the person of Jesus.

The OT law said to not steal or covet; Jesus said to give freely to the poor. The OT law said don't murder; Jesus said to love our enemies. The OT law said to sacrifice cattle, bulls and sheep to God; Jesus called us to be living sacrifices. The OT law said to commit no adultery; Jesus says to love our spouses as ourselves. The OT law said to not worship lifeless idols; Jesus invited us to true life for free. The OT law said to honor our parents; Jesus said to take them into our homes

---

[11] James 4:6

[12] These words were first coined together by Dr. Mark and Patti Virkler in their book *Rivers of Grace* in the context of the OT's importance and is used with permission.

to help us, and care for them. The OT law said to not work on the Sabbath; Jesus said don't be greedy and it is healthy to do good on the Sabbath. The OT law said not to use the Lord's Name in vain; Jesus says we get to call God our Father. The OT law said, "An eye for an eye, and a tooth for a tooth," but Jesus said use non-violence to spread love. The OT law said bear no false witness; Jesus said to speak the truth in love, believe the best about people, and not to judge or condemn others. The OT law said to give a percentage of what you had; Jesus asks us to be generous just like He is.

Holding obsessively onto laws to somehow let them save me from sin, inevitably sucks the life and joy out of me. However, little "t" truths set me free like an uncaged bird; but if I hold onto these truths or books that contain them too tightly and religiously, (including this one) they too start to suck the life out of me. When it comes to truth, I need the *big* "T" Truth, Jesus Christ. He will supply, in many ways, the right little "t" truths at the right times—with the right touch and enough grace, when I am open to them and listening for them.

Any commandment given by Jesus, that seems grossly unfair to me, must not be carried about like a burdensome negative weight. Instead I choose to trust Jesus, and that He will help me carry it out at the appropriate times. My faith is in Jesus saving me, not in laws saving me, no matter how good the laws are. I love because I care, not because I want to execute a law.

The law was made for those who sin; by that I mean the law only points out our sins. The law can't save us from our sins; only Jesus can save us from our sins.

Jesus lifts us up to supernatural love through prayer. By this I mean that after we have repented in prayer from a sin in question, we should ask Jesus to lift us up to supernatural love in that area believing Him for it. And, then walking in that grace in trust that Jesus keeps His promises to answer our prayers. This is the meaning of walking in grace. These periods of walking in grace may be short lived at first if we have a lot of repenting to do. But don't give up! There is so much waiting for each of us!

Focusing On Jesus

Once I get healthy in an area because the corresponding little "t" truth has done its job, then I don't need to focus on it anymore until I need it again. I don't keep taking a certain cough medicine when I no longer have a cold. My focus and attention ought to be redirected to Jesus and His grace and not at the little "t" truths that have set me free in certain areas.

It is about the Grace Giver, and His grace flows into me naturally, if I don't block it with my pride. And if I don't block it, then it will flow into my life and out of me into all those people I am called to love—both friends and enemies.

When I have had wonderful insights it has been easy to get preachy. And I know that many times God has spoken to me indirectly through people, but it often does not clue into my mind immediately that what was spoken applies to me. I think this is true of others too. The Holy Spirit is a far better convincer about sin than we are. He does not do so to make us feel judged, and remain guilty, shamed and condemned, but to have a change of heart, and to joyously go our way thereafter.

Criticizing people when we have our own blind spots is hypocritical, unloving, and hurtful—and should be abandoned. We are not moral policemen. Thankfully, God loves us so much that He does all in His power to convince us to choose healthy attitudes instead.

When I pray, "God, please help 'so and so' be *more like me* in this area of love or humility," I am being proud and judgmental. I ought not to compare myself with others, put them down, and attempt to raise myself up in prayer. No one has arrived. When I do grow in love and humility I give glory to God. Let me not pretend that I am a paragon of virtue or have it all together.

We all have gaps in our thinking, reasoning, understanding, and philosophies; and we all fall short in our actions to love and be completely humble in every area of our lives. All of us to some degree major on minor issues, and we all minor on some major issues. We skip over stuff that ought to be done when people are not looking because we think we can get away with it. We cannot judge or condemn other people; the Sermon on the Mount teaches[13] us to not judge or condemn others no matter how informed we think we are.

The tools outlined in this book are basic but not always easy to apply. Using them in relationship with Jesus, through prayer, is slowly making me spiritually healthy. And I ought not to think I have mastered humility once a victory or string of victories is achieved.

Law vs. Grace

When the Bible calls for honest, confessional prayer it is not asking the child of God to view God's throne room as a court of law. It is asking us to look at His throne room as a family room. The difference is that the law mentality deals only with not wanting to go to Hell (which can be a very selfish preoccupation for some), whereas the family room attitude has to do with admitting how we hurt or wronged people, or grieved God's heart. But more than that, it is where we seek healing in ourselves and our relationships, and where we want forgiveness in our lives and for those who did the hurting. This isn't done to bring about shame, humiliation, fear, self-pity, anger, judgment, or condemnation. It is diagnostic in nature and is meant to bring healing to self-wounds and relationship-wounds through God's grace and loving touch. The law approach does not do this. The law approach just cares whether you are guilty or not and what your penance and sentence will be.

---

[13] Cf. Matthew 7:1-6

The law approach is only concerned about heaven and hell whereas the grace approach considers that but is much more. Grace is interested in restorative justice; the healing in the here and now of the hurting self, broken relationships, and hurting people. Grace is holistic and closer to the heart of Father God. God is not a cold judge but a warm restorer.

The law approach has no humor, joy, freshness, life, or imagination associated with it, because it is only concerned about the outcome. The grace approach does embrace humor, joy, warmth, freshness, life, and imagination, because it is not a "heaven vs. hell" approach but an "unhealthy vs. healthy" approach to life. There is no condemnation for those in Christ Jesus.[14]

The way I talk to God is the way I will talk with others, so changing my attitudes in prayer will give deeper intimacy with God as well as more warmth towards people.

Many people view the context of confessing sin to God as a court of law affair—they see confessing sin and seeking repentance, as the way to get right with God and nullify one's fears of going to Hell. Many other people (myself included) view confessing sin to God and seeking to repent from sin, as the way to get rid of guilt and become free of the intrinsic consequences of sin that lead to death and Hell. They see getting clean as the way to heal their relationships with God and others. Such people view meeting with God as set in a family room, because there is now no condemnation for those who are in Christ Jesus.

Serious and not so serious sins do separate us from God; the former in big ways and the latter in smaller ways. Either way, we need to seek forgiveness to get right with God, and with His grace seek repentance. If we are not right with God, then sin's intrinsic consequences will, more and more, be visited on us daily. And in such cases we are playing with fire.

The more we push God away, the more we invite death and Hell—even experiencing it here on earth and in our lives.

The court of law people only see repentance as something that frees them from Hell. Whereas the family room people see repentance more as something that comes out of seeking healthy relationships with God and others, rather than attempting to appease an angry God and other people. If we do not love people, we don't love God.

Difficulties of Transformation

In my experience, the process of transformation can be difficult. It begins with promises and preparation, but then life gradually gets more frustrating and counter intuitive. It comes to a point where the difficulties are so extreme that it seems absurd that things will change. You believe the promises, but your mind may disagree with your faith in your heart. Things can just seem so unfair, while demons lie to you saying "God isn't good." Eventually, self-pity becomes

---

[14] Cf. Romans 8:1

an option—and if indulged in, and not repented from—it can rob one of the blessings that are promised. In some cases, people jettison their faith because the wait is too long, and that is *really* sad! But when we come to understand and master our self-pity through grace and truth, we will inherit the promises.

Jesus Heals Our Pain

Pain alone does not in itself make one humble or heal. When pain is with us our reactions to it can be negative (bitter, proud, envious, self-pitying) and that can lead to being demanding (judgmental, angry, hostile, rebellious, hateful, resentful), with cries of unfairness. But God can use pain to prepare us for healing, if we choose to humble ourselves in its presence.

It is faith in Jesus that brings spiritual healing and cleansing from sins through spiritual medicines. And it is faith that helps me get through the pain that accompanies the surgery He wants to perform on me. I just need to know how to access the medicines; and I do so through praying God's promises (found in Holy Scripture) in strategic ways. I do not let self-pity rob me of the treasures awaiting me.

Truth sets people free. Jesus is our Savior, not pain. Pain can alert us to the need of a Savior. Pain happens as we rub shoulders with real life and struggle to grow spiritually, seemingly without success. But Jesus waits patiently for us to turn to him. It is how we navigate pain that can bring blessings; for it is the Savior of the world, Jesus, who heals, forgives and cleanses us, not the pain. Let's not give up when seeking spiritual healing! It starts with prayer that says God is good and a rewarder of those who seek Him. Seeking God with a demanding spirit that stems from self-pity is unhealthy, but seeking God to get rid of self-pity is healthy.

I view the principles, promises, and truths in this book as prescriptions and medicines to get me healthy; I try to be serious about them and I try to understand them. But at the same time I try not to forget the face of Jesus—His warmth, kindness, grace, patience, love, compassion, and tears of joy and sadness. He is with me all the way. Keeping my sense of humor has been very important. There is joy in the journey.

It is so easy to acquire sour attitudes, but wholesome ones seem so much harder to get. But I am the only one who can change my attitudes, with Jesus' help, once I understand what their functions are.

As the saying goes the journey to wholeness is a marathon, not a sprint. There are periods in life where we encounter all sorts of chaos, pain, random acts of cruelty, and senseless suffering. This can confuse us, can make us question the goodness of God, and can trigger a reaction of self-pity in us. Only by focusing on the goal, and focusing on the grace, truths, and promises of God will we be able to make it through the messiness of life. Without a goal, or a healthy focus we are more susceptible to the lies of the devil; he will do whatever is in his power to torment us, neutralize us, and draw us away from the straight and narrow path before us.

The methods I use to repent and renew my mind in this book are dogmatically systematic, and can be looked at as cold algorithms, but I refuse to look at them and follow them that way. Staying open to the Holy Trinity speaking to me, and trying not to conform to cold methods is where I have had the most success. I look at the principles in this book as medicines that bring healing, but they all have limitations.

The attitudes of fear, pride, coveting, jealousy, using people, compulsive-laziness, compulsive-indulging, greed, selfishness, judging... etc. all promise things they can't give me. Even though they are my enemies, I find myself agreeing with them when it is convenient. Undoing the lies through which the devils make their promises is key to winning these battles, and requires renewing my mind. Fighting off temptation, seeking progress, and not letting things get me bogged down are important to the day-to-day process of not stagnating. Killing the attitudes of self-pity (that can lead to ugly demanding), bitterness, conceit, resentments, jealousy, and anger helps us to win and occupy the Promised Land.

Truth is so very important. We are confronted with so much misrepresentation in our daily lives; media lies about 'the good life', 'money is king', entrenched prejudices and so forth, with Bible truths spurned or ignored. My response to people who confidently assert these kind of things as truth should not be to try to correct them when they have not asked for my advice, but to use healthy wisdom with respect and without judgment, in how I relate with them.

In this book, very specific categories of sin will be pointed out, making up the roots, branches, and fruits of the old life within me—"the tree of knowledge of good and evil"—and will be shown to be connected. Being able to pray through them to God in logical and systematic ways helped to dismantle this old structure, and established new outlets for grace to bear love in my relational life.

When I confess my sins to God as part of the processes described in this book I have found from experience that the peace granted through forgiveness ought to *really* be savored, reflected on, appreciated, and accepted, as gifts made possible because of Jesus' crucifixion and resurrection. This gift of peace stabilizes me, calms me down, and allows God's grace to flow through me more perfectly. I don't rush or intellectualize the process of being forgiven, because God's felt presence is very real. In following this wisdom, I eventually got in touch with the joy of my salvation. I strongly encourage you to not abandon the emotional aspects when confessing one's sins to Him.

The Twelve-Principles

Generally, the process of inner transformation, described in this book involves the following daily principles that I practice:

1. Pursue a relationship with God through faith in Jesus with His grace that results in a love that grows for God and people and ourselves.

2. Refuse to wallow in self-pity, "poor me" thinking and believing God to be unfair. Refuse to attack, criticize or judge God when things seem upside down. Do not mistaken loyalty to God as a sign that you aren't holding any resentments against Him.

3. Ceaselessly pray (see Chapter 4). This enables me to find my bearings and journey with God in faith.

4. Ask the Holy Spirit to heal my mind and heart regularly. Like when I'm in distress feeling self-pity and have a mean attitude accompanying my anger that prevents me from loving those people I meet daily.

5. Give up pretending that I don't have the wounds I have. Be honest and choose to humble myself with faith in Jesus. Stop doing life on my own terms. Stop pushing bad stuff down or shoving it under carpets. Learn to process your baggage in your mind and heart (with the strategies found in this book).

6. Become aware of the connections found in "The Tree of Knowledge of Good and Evil" diagram found in this book (that in shorthand I may simply call the Tree Diagram). And realize that the foolish sins, judgments, criticisms, and condemning attitudes that we have that get triggered in certain contexts in certain relationships aren't just past sins but they help form the sin-structure within. We ask God to open our eyes to the whole sin-structure that is hidden within us in the form of the Tree Diagram. This doesn't happen all at once. It is a journey; not an eternity.

7. When you see stuff in the present that looks like it relates to stuff from the past that wasn't dealt with wisely. Then look at the parts in Tree Diagram that seem to connect the foolish past with the unhealthy-compulsive-triggered-present. Then construct a Sin-Anatomy Table with the help of the Holy Spirit by using a Sin-Conduit Structure from the Tree Diagram that is appropriate. Don't do it with a mean, ugly, angry and judgmental energy. Love God and your neighbors as yourself: kindly and caringly. Get in touch with your remorse for your sins.

8. Speak to God about the connections in your Sin-Conduit Structure that helps determine any Sin-Anatomy Tables you might have. Ask Jesus for guidance and search within yourself with His light. Don't rush things. Ask Jesus simple questions and listen to the spontaneous thoughts that come your way. Don't be critical or hard on yourself and others. If you get confusing communications when speaking with God, then you need to draw back and re-shape your questions with Jesus' help through faith and grace. Confusion I have learned results from mixing a wise approach somehow with an unhealthy approach at the same time and this causes the confusion.

9. After moving from "The Tree of Knowledge of Good and Evil" diagram to a certain Sin-Conduit Structure to a specific Sin-Anatomy Table. Then it is time to confess accurately, gently, contritely and genuinely the sins in the Sin-Anatomy Table to God. Don't embellish or minimize the weight of your sins. Just be honest, kind, caring and open to correction.

10. Then repent in faith in prayer with Jesus' help and grace from the sins and unhealthy attitudes you confessed to God in the previous step found in the corresponding Sin-Anatomy Table you made with Jesus' help.

11. Renew your mind (see Chapter 4 for advice). Ask God to give you the wisdom that unshackles the lies you believed that gave "The Tree of Knowledge of Good and Evil Within You" its dark power to grow and mutilate the image of God you were created in. Listen to God and those people He sends into your life with truth and Godly wisdom.

12. Choose to submit to God by being obedient to His Commands that are summed up in: "Do unto others as you wish them to do to you" with clean energy and resist the tendency to coast in the flesh and indulge in earthly pleasures. Make restitution and apologize without hurting or harming anyone we hurt or harmed in the past.

These Twelve-Principles form the nucleus of this book. The Twelve-Principles above will help one get spiritually healthy and to bear the fruit of the Holy Spirit. Be sure to look up working definitions of terms when given, as without them this book has no power to change anyone. The principles above will be used and/ or discussed in depth in this book, in the context of dismantling "the tree of knowledge of good and evil" within me. I will attempt to explain my take on these basics of the Christian life (which I did not understand well or did not know the importance of for a very long time) that need to be practiced daily to remain free to love God, oneself, and one's neighbors. They are the basics to growing up into maturity, deep fellowship with people, and intimacy with God. They are done through Jesus' grace and truth—not self-righteous self-effort.

Principles 6-12 are strongly connected to the three diagrams below. The process of inner transformation in this book involves becoming familiar with how "the tree of knowledge of good and evil" functions in our lives via this Sin Diagram:

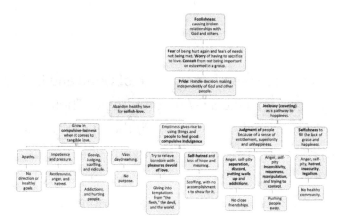

And becoming aware of particular Sin-Conduit Structures in one's life as may be indicated here:

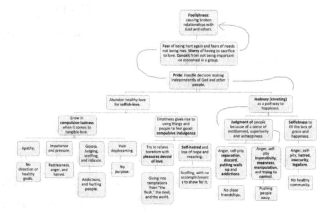

That leads us to understanding the Sin-Conduit Structure in the form of a Sin-Anatomy Table that looks something like:

Meanness & Intolerance towards others	Judging	Coveting & Jealousy	Pride	Fear	Foolishness
	<=	<=	<=	<=	<= Cause and Effect
I want my will done (and I choose to do it meanly) instead of aiming for God's will to be done through me: i.e. "that I obey the Golden Rule".	Subconsciously or consciously I demanded: "An eye for an eye, and a tooth for a tooth" treatment towards those in my way... And I actually wanted karma visited on these people instead of grace.	I wanted to get my desires fulfilled ASAP demanding that others cooperate with me so I can get my way.	I see myself as the center of the universe. So my desires are more important than other people's.	I might have to get my hands dirty and love people other than myself. Believing the lie: "Loving people is too hard and unimportant".	People matter only insofar as they help me out with my chosen causes. I am committed to feeling as little pain as possible.
When I treated so and so disrespectfully...					
Confession & Repenting in Faith =>	=>	=>	=>	=>	

That tells a story on how certain strongholds developed. We can confess such Sin-Anatomy Tables to God in detail, repent in prayer from the sins found in them with Jesus help, so that we can begin to renew our minds/ hearts. This brings healthy relational-freedom into our lives as the strongholds get dismantled.

There are many details and suggested methods of prayer that come with these diagrams in this book. Praying with wrong energy and postures builds Satan's kingdom not God's. Thankfully the Holy Spirit will never leave us nor forsake us and leads us into the truth and supernatural love.

Freedom is found in being who we were originally created to be and are recreated to be through Christ Jesus, not conforming to rules or ideals with pressure.

When we are renewing our minds confusion will be a visitor. That means we need to often find our bearings because we need some clarity of mind. We need to embrace healthy energy to process our divided loyalties, emotions, attitudes, beliefs, thinking, understanding, and knowledge when it comes to our relationships. We make this spiritual progress in prayer, and not through analyzing.

Renewing our minds means learning to see God, others, and ourselves positively, healthily, gracefully, and warmly. Sour, negative, judgmental attitudes can and should be removed from our relationships by embracing the Golden Rule with grace and Jesus commands in the NT. In getting free from our negative sinful attitudes we will have a foretaste of Heaven on earth. But we need to accept life as a bumpy journey, and people as perfectly imperfect too.

When it comes to lies we sometimes believe them because we trust their source, or foolishly see them as true because they have just enough truth to sway us. Asking the Holy Spirit to heal our hearts and minds, to show us what needs to be thrown away, and to lead us into the truth—and believing He will—is key to finding renewal in our thinking. We then need to focus on loving others and at the same time listening for little "t" truths to guide and set us free. We know something is true when it sets us free.

Live By Grace Thinking

We aim to live by grace thinking and not by law thinking when seeking to love or being tempted to sin. Grace is activated when I ask Jesus for it and receive it by faith, not only at the moment of salvation, but in every situation and every moment.

We make the most of every opportunity, and give our lives to something greater than ourselves—namely God. And out of caring obedience to Jesus, carry out His commands through grace and truth, via His teachings, and in the light of His promises (i.e. practice the Golden Rule in the context of grace).

Grace thinking means we focus on caring for people and not on rules or principles so much. Rules can often dehumanize people, especially when there is something in it for us and resonates with "I'm the center of the universe" thinking. So as we approach each day, there are so many good things we can do instead of focusing on rules all of the time; choosing the right things to do requires two-way communication with God through journaling.

We always return our focus to Jesus. Choose to let Jesus save us through trust in Him. Remind ourselves often that it is Jesus who saves us from sin and enables us to love.

We go deeper when feeling guilty, perplexed, or confused. We seek God with all our hearts and embrace His love and peace. We deal with any unpleasantness through relationship with Jesus and through His truth and grace. We choose to believe there is more that God has in store for us, always returning to the basics of Christianity to tackle the giants in the Promised Land. Basics like humility, confession, repentance, renewing the mind, faith, hope, and Love.

Realize we are not alone in our struggles, weaknesses, and challenges. Jesus is with us to help, direct, and protect us. This comes from the promise of His grace, which means His empowering presence is with us always; no matter how dark it gets, there is always hope. This has the ability to bring real peace and focus, removing many battles God does not intend us to fight, like struggling with compulsions to sin or powerlessness to love. This is crucial to tapping into the person of Jesus: To believe We are not alone and that Jesus is with us now and always makes us strong.

We practice prayer in the forms of making petitions, seeking instruction, worshipping God, and developing our friendships with Him through journaling.

We view life as a learning curve; view failures as part of one's learning curve and as doorways to seeing things in new, healthy, and positive ways. This keeps one from getting discouraged and full of self-pity.

Just when things seem to get good they can get really bad. The last lap is always the most difficult. This is meant as a lesson that life isn't always going to be easy; that we must put our full armor on and be ready for whatever comes: the good, the bad, and the ugly.

Once a certain stronghold is totally dismantled, then one can claim the healthy freedom Jesus promised, and to see oneself as a new creation in that context[15]. This new identity ought to be claimed, and then to move from one's head outwards to active love in one's relationships. If one does not move out of the head, then the devil will continually argue with you and attack you in order to neutralize you and your freedom will be fleeting and may eventually vanish. Truth doesn't just change what we believe, but our identities.

Connecting With God Through Prayer

When we realize we have sinful thoughts, the first thing to do is to connect with God; dialogue and reason with Him in prayer to get our bearings straight. We should not blindly mechanically, fearfully, or religiously confess our "supposed" sins immediately. Not all thoughts in our heads are ours. The healthiest thing to do is talk with the Holy Spirit as our friend and guardian, and if He says it is okay, then go ahead and confess the unhealthy thoughts that spring from our unhealthy attitudes.

It is not wise to jump to conclusions when praying about the vices mentioned here. Trying to not fall for red herrings is wise, although as beginners that will happen as part of the learning curves we are on. The understanding drawn from the Tree Diagram is a skeletal framework meant to

---

[15] Cf. 2 Corinthians 5:17

help bring healing. But the rooted motives and intrigues of the heart need to be searched out with a commitment to truth, respect, wisdom, and God's leading will—not with judgment, hatred, pressure on oneself, or trying to conform to rules. Confusion around hurts or wounds needs to be walked through into the light, or attacked skillfully with practical wisdom and God's empowering presence and leading. God is with us in this process.

Situations have arisen in the past that seemed to have many possible courses of healing through many seemingly wise prayers. And I would try praying some of them only to find out that I didn't see the whole picture. I felt numb and carnal inside instead of feeling free. I found I had unwisely trampled on stuff somehow with unhealthy prayers of mine. I needed to be more connected, observant, and aware of what I was doing, and then address the issues in my heart or relationships from a healthier perspective led by God. Having said this, it can be hit-and-miss at times when it comes to praying healthily and making progress. But I learned over time to refrain from generalizing and rushing over details in prayer and when making resolutions.

I have felt numbness and carnal energy within me in the following circumstances:

1. Confessing a sin over and over, that was already forgiven and dealt with is not healthy or wise, as it is not genuine and respectful of the truth that God already forgave. Prayer should not be lazy, cavalier, or insulated from the truth. But it is healthy to persevere in praying about sin that seemingly doesn't want to go away. Aim to go deeper in prayer each time to eventually get rid of all the roots and bad fruit.
2. Praying to God with a proud attitude instead of approaching God to get rid of my pride.
3. Using prayer like a spell, an algorithm, or a coin we put into a vending machine to get what we want, instead of humbly respecting that God's will be done.
4. Making self-righteous declarations or independent commitments to correct behaviors in and even out of prayer.
5. Having a mean and angry tone in prayer, when seeking change, fueled by a judgmental, "I'm not like those other people," self-righteous attitude.
6. Making huge blanketed prayers that sweep sins, feelings, motivations, energies, and attitudes under rugs, rather than being real and in touch with what is within me. Blankets obscure details, and details involve lies or truths that if not dealt with limit what God can do in us. Truth sets us free.
7. Praying an acceptable prayer that God could use to start processing the "bad stuff" and clean me up inside, but nothing happening because I won't relax and allow Him do what I asked. For example, when I push "bad stuff" down inside me instead of connecting with it and cooperating with God to process it. This stops me from doing healthy business with God.

When I find myself in these situations I have learned that it is wise for me to confess what went wrong, give it up in faith, ask for the opposite virtue, trust in Jesus' presence, and walk forward believing grace and truth are restoring and guiding me (we walk by faith and not sight).

Example of Conflict With Another Person

For instance, I might think I need to forgive a person for holding back on something I wanted, but the real issue can be that I have a demanding, coveting, and grasping spirit that is rooted in pride and selfishness. If it is the latter, then no amount of forgiving the other person will heal the relationship, but when I confess to God the sin in my heart, and repent in prayer I will find healing and love in me for the person who was seemingly holding out on me.

On the other hand, the situation could be reversed; it might have nothing to do with my pride or supposed jealousy, but that the other person was insensitive towards me. In this case, I need to forgive them from the heart so I can continue to love them.

The situation can perhaps involve hypocritical expectations on my part, with there being dirty laundry belonging to the other party too. This should be sorted out with wisdom and prayer.

I might have believed lies about the people involved or even myself; either way the Holy Spirit needs to be invited into the situation. I need to listen and obey. I need to know when to sit back and wait for wisdom and when to fight. To fight off any oppressing thoughts that cause confusion with lies or accusations in my mind. To fight so my moral compass, intuition, and conscience can once again speak to me, so I will know where I stand and what to do.

I might not have the full picture so I need to give the benefit of the doubt to all the people involved, as love believes the best about people.

When conflicts arise I need to own my anger. I might direct my anger one way only to find out it should have been directed another way. That is par for the course. That does not mean the anger shouldn't have existed—it is a sign that something is wrong, although I might not know the details or reasons for it immediately. I need to try to not jump to harmful conclusions and actions. I need to focus on nonviolent conflict resolution when the anger signal has gone off—if I do this, then my anger has done its job. I need courage to confront people only when I am levelheaded and when needed, provided the Lord gives the go ahead.

When I first started working the Tree Diagram found in this book, I was dealing with generalities and mostly unhealthy attitudes rooted in the past. This was difficult because my memory was not always reliable. After quite some time, I began to learn how to navigate situations in real time more wisely, because I was able to get rid of baggage or distorted lens strategies I developed. These situations in the present became more hopeful than before to deal with because of the healthy relational wisdom I was able to learn from Jesus on how to navigate my relationships. I see more options now: I am getting a better feel for how healthy relationships work; I am learning how to diffuse conflicts in healthy nonviolent ways; and I am understanding how to give opinions that are not insulting. This all leads to gentleness, humility, and love.

Gentleness does not mean I don't own my anger, because if I don't own my anger and process it healthily, then my gentleness is fake. The processes outlined in this book, when implemented, also leads to greater intimacy: relating on deeper levels, being more honest with people, sharing warmer humor. I no longer rely on attitudes of self-pity, anger or meanness (because of little disappointments), demand things or use force to get things.

Sometimes something can hit me the wrong way and I think it is a momentary thing, yet it negatively affects my thinking, attitudes, and the way I navigate relationships until it is processed in a healthy way. Not processing the baggage can cause me to engage in plenty of self-pity and angry pressure because that may be part of my strategy to attempt fixing things spiritually. But this is no way to get to the place of living out the Golden Rule in my life. I feel restricted, clumsy, powerless, and disconnected when this happens. And it is not that I'm screaming for blood, or want revenge—I'm just *really* slow in realizing that I took offense, or hold things against other people at times. In sharing this with others I know I'm not the only one who experiences such things. Things are getting healthier over time though.

My feelings can still linger around a bit. And they linger because I often say to myself, "Because I still sort of feel them they must be my true state," and so it validates my "old self." This is dangerous and untrue. When we see movies, we will see stories portrayed as true that we naturally get emotional about even though it is all being acted out; likewise the attitudes I experience don't mean the beliefs behind them are always true or are grounded in reality. When thoughts enter our heads they immediately trigger our emotions and we experience them whether or not they are true or false. It is important to me to not struggle with them in a dark way, and to not wrestle with them in my own negative energy trying to make negative, uncomfortable emotions vanish.

It is not a good idea to navigate purely by my feelings, or attempt to manufacture feelings by my own strength to feel holy, pure, or happy. Feelings fluctuate, and truth is a better compass. Having said this, feelings (emotions, energies, attitudes) generated by using people, pride, coveting, jealousy, selfishness, self-pity, anger, conceit, fear, and judging should be monitored by what thoughts trigger them at the time. And if I don't want the feelings generated by these vices, I have learned that I must deal with my beliefs and thinking in the context of "the tree of knowledge of good and evil" within, as outlined in this book (through prayer, renewing the mind and heart, and through a relationship with Jesus).

The maxim: "the universal needs to be made particular" always applies to the Golden Rule. But when I can't seem to focus on or practice the Golden Rule then it can be quite the fight. I might need to forgive people I am holding resentments towards; I might need to accept my emotions (i.e. anger) and process them in prayer using "I" statements; I might need to move from judging people to truth telling and grace. Sometimes asking the Holy Spirit to heal my mind and waiting for His touch might be all I can do. He will always come through.

I have realized that my identity should not be that of a "slave" or to see myself as a perpetual victim to the whims, assaults, violations, disappointments, negativity, and shortcomings coming from others. When experiencing negative emotions, it is so easy to start having negative cynical thoughts that are not based in reality, but inspired by feelings that have nothing to do with what is contextually happening.

I can have positive attitudes in the face of devastating news. I can choose to be cheerful when people expect more from me than I was counting on. My emotions and attitudes don't have to be at the mercies of capricious circumstances, fickle or selfish people, or honest people who are just doing their thing. I don't have to have a victim mentality. I can own and process my attitudes, reactions and emotions, in response to disagreeable things, for they determine the difference between being strong in joy and weak in self-pity. It is the difference between peace and unhealthily processed anger. I can be joyful so much more than Satan wants me to think I can. I don't want to go by my feelings, but by the truth and God's unconditional love! Doing this stabilizes me.

I make progress when Jesus confronts my perfectionist tendencies with liberating truths. Perfectionism makes me hard on myself and others. The law expects complete compliance, but I'm not the law, so I can choose to be gracious instead like God is. Practicing "do to others as I want done to me" gives me more connection to what I personally desire, and to want the best for others too.

The war against pride is constant; the battles are the only possible victories. There are usually other sins involved with the attitudes of pride, coveting, jealousy, using people, judgments, selfishness, compulsive-laziness, and compulsive-indulging. They must all be processed if I want freedom to love others deeply. Self-pity is an attitude that can grow so quickly when things don't go a person's way, and I have learned that it is often the first issue that needs to be dealt with, together with my anger. Also, it is not wise to box things in or compartmentalize stuff. For instance, my insensitivity and meanness have been the results of pride, jealousy, and judging; but insensitivity and meanness also need to be confessed together with the pride, jealousy, and judging in prayer for there to be victory and progress in the spiritual journey. The confessional prayers I have learned need to be accurate, gentle, heartfelt and said with the same intensity as the vices and sinful attitudes I have participated in. I also need to repent in prayer from these vices and sinful attitudes when aware of them.

Shallow prayer does not work or get to the roots of spiritual maladies. Just saying "no" to sins is not enough. I must aim high enough to replace the darkness with light for there to be real lasting change. Jesus provides this. Going deeper is a wise strategy when it comes to growth.[16]

---

[16] Advice from my friend Alex Angioli.

4 How I've Learnt To Dismantle The Tree Of Knowledge Of Good And Evil Within Me

The "tree of knowledge of good and evil" diagram spoken about here and the theology found in this book have helped me tackle my sin strongholds within, through strategic prayer. This structure is not meant to be analyzed in a vacuum devoid of God's input. Knowledge of the structure of "the tree of knowledge of good and evil" is intended to facilitate questions that I am able to ask God, about relating to my history and current story. The answers lead to confession, repentance, and forgiveness in order to dismantle the tree so that love can thrive within me. Once the sin strongholds from the tree are dismantled, one's thinking, and habits needs to be tackled next[17]. We know when this happens because the compulsions are gone. We see the lies for what they are, but we don't automatically know how to think healthily and can still be confused. This makes sense, because the tree structure that we removed, with God's help, did dry up the soil where it was planted in our hearts. The part of one's heart affected needs to be tilled, seeded with Scripture, and watered with the Holy Spirit. And we need to spend time in prayer with Jesus so He can speak life into our parched, desert like hearts.

All journeys of healing, made possible by God, begin with and are sustained by a faith that says that God is good and trustworthy. The Gospel of Luke says about some sick men who met Jesus that "they were healed as they went on their way."[18] This is the way it is with most healing; it takes time— repeatedly going deeper in prayer. I believe what the Holy Spirit communicates to me; to get rid of my self-pity, doubt, pettiness, unbelief, accusations, attacks, judgments, anger, demanding nature, inflexibility, and "it's unfair to wait so long" thinking, directed negatively at God and those I fail to love. Instead the Holy Spirit asks that I learn how to abide in Jesus through faith and with a teachable attitude, so God is able to get the healing process going.

Jesus is the True Vine and I need to put my faith in Him, if I want to grow in bearing good fruit. I can't earn a spot in the true Vine by my actions, piety, holiness, human intellect, positions, degrees, or great philosophies. I can't earn a good relationship with God. By resting in Jesus through grace and faith I will, if I am committed to mercy, bear much good fruit, and in the process dismantle the dead tree structure within me.

The "tree of knowledge of good and evil" promises to keep me in control and "special"; it has a devilish "understanding" and "energy belief structure" of supposed goodness that bears the bad

---

[17] In coming to grips with my faulty understanding on love and pride, I wrote two more books titled *Exploring Faith, Hope & Love,* and *Contrasting Humility and Pride* respectively.
[18] Luke 17:14

fruit that sane people "really" don't want in their lives.

In becoming aware of the connections between the building blocks from "the tree of knowledge of good and evil," it is best to look at my bad fruit and ask God and myself what active or reactive sins I participated in. These sins can perhaps occur when hurts, possible foolish beliefs and fears, materialized in traumatic moments or conflicts from my past. Once the connections are understood and hit home, then I have found it is time to dismantle them through grace, truth, strategic prayer, confession, repentance, forgiveness, conquering fears, and renewing one's mind (working upwards through the Tree Diagram presented earlier using the correct Sin-Conduit Structures). In constructing these Sin-Anatomy tables I have found the process to go more smoothly and deeply. This keeps the guessing and frustration to a minimum, and helps me find and dismantle the real motivations and roots for my sin strongholds in less time. And therefore I grow in the freedom to love with each victory.

When confusion and carnal energy operate in the present, know that the past may not fully be dealt with—especially when it comes to one's greatest hurts and wounds. These wounds occur when the devil promises things that seemed justified, however, the devil's promises are always empty and rob people of their true humanity.

Intense fear and confusion go together. They can cloud one's judgment into believing that one has the power and control. But when the power and control comes from the dark side i.e. in the situation of fear and confusion the devil tries to justify everyone's sense of injustice or unfairness to win them over to permanent resentments. This needs to be prayed through thoroughly for healing and freedom to flourish and thrive, by forgiving the agents of our hurts and learning to believe the real truth about what happened, and how to "really" approach life.

Below is my "tree of the knowledge of good and evil" within. I have learned to "work out my salvation" by dismantling it and its influence within me through confession, repentance in prayer, renewing my mind, giving up fears, and forgiving. I do so based on what is currently happening in my life spiritually, by noticing the triggers and the bad fruit involved. I work my way up the Tree Diagram in prayer, noticing my emotions and what I'm after and dealing with one stronghold after another, until I get to the source: sins, resentments and fears that spring from making judgments on hurts that I justified by believing foolish lies. Yes, some building blocks like anger appear in a lot of places in the Tree Diagram, but understanding the theme, the emotions, and the contexts of one's sins helps locate the correct Sin-Conduit Structure to be dealt with. Healing possible wounds in my heart, such as forgiving resentments or giving up judgments about people, is wise. For instance, if I struggle with apathy, then I can pray through the connections from the bottom upwards (the lighter arrow-line shown in the diagram below). I go from sin to sin or attitude to attitude until I deal with my wounds, foolishness, and fears. In so doing I cooperate with God in healing my broken heart through His grace and truth. I have also made my relationships with others healthier by working this process out thoroughly.

When searching for Sin-Conduit Structures to eventually dismantle in prayer. We look at our sins located at the bottom of the Tree Diagram and ask what themes are presented in each scenario. The most obvious themes are: "Coveting/jealousy, judgment, selfishness, abandoning love, compulsive-laziness, and compulsive-indulging." To me they are the most visible themes when I have sinned (my conscience usually tells me quickly enough). And, by reflection I see the connections between the branches of sins all the way up to the top through to my pride, my fears, and the roots: my foolishly broken relationships with God and others (either done in the past or established in the present). If this does not work because of too much confusion then it is always easier to ask God which building blocks form the sin-conduit in question one block at a time. This helps to give confidence that one is on track. Praying from the bottom up through the relevant connections will bring healing and growth. Because life is messy and complicated, I am working these connections in prayer regularly over time. And I am slowly growing in purity of heart as God promises in Revelation 3:18, by inviting grace and truth into my life through relationship and two-way prayer with Jesus.

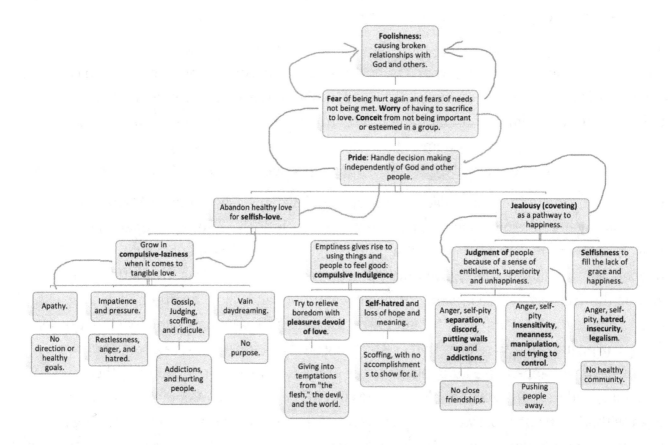

For example (following the dark-arrow line), in the past, I had somebody withholding something that I used to take for granted. I felt hurt and angry because it had been denied. I was therefore tempted to *try to control* the person with my anger, because I was jealous that they withheld something from me but were still giving it to others. This was connected to unhealthy *pride*, because I judged the person in a negative light thinking I knew better than them; but then the pride is connected to the *fear* of losing forever what was being withheld. The way I dealt with this is to pray through the connections in a thorough manner. Something like this:

> Lord God, I confess that I am angry with this person and want to control them real badly so I'll get what I want: "their friendship" that they are now withholding from me. I confess that this is my sense of entitlement and jealousy coming out. I regret this, and ask for your forgiveness. I give up with your help in faith Lord Jesus, meanly wanting to demand their warmth, and wanting to control them, and selfishly wanting to make things my way out of jealousy. I admit this all comes from my pride that says I know best, and things should revolve around me instead. I have approached things this way because I fear losing this person. I give up this pride and fear with your help in faith Lord Jesus. Lord God, I confess that I have a history of wanting to force my friendships onto others and I give up this flawed way of using people right now. Thank you for forgiving me, and healing me from this now Lord Jesus. I will now renew my mind with your truth and grace knowing you are not coercive in nature, and so I don't want to be either. Thank you and Amen.

The reason why this method works is because it connects the mind and the heart with God in a biblical, thorough, and inside-out, strategic way. It deals with many of the roots and growths that have lived in me, bringing spiritual death into my life over the years.

Praying repeatedly in this way, in the different contexts of my relational life, is helping to slowly dismantle the strongholds mentioned in the Tree Diagram. My confession and prayer needs to be genuine, and so I will define these terms in ways that work for me. This is not a complete map to freedom; I know that other truths are needed to heal our hearts so we can love people more deeply over time. There may be more branches, so going deeper in prayer is wise if things keep getting triggered from the present.

There are times when I become aware of unhealthy things that I don't know how to label or classify and therefore deal with. I have found that when I experience these things there are two strategies I can employ.

1. Ask God to show me what I'm not seeing and wait on Him to bring to mind what He wants me to pray about.
2. Connect with the feelings, unhealthy attitudes, or energies and pray to God asking Him, "What am I feeling inside Lord Jesus?" Then wait and search for spontaneous words, which come from the Holy Spirit, that describe the energy.

The second method is wisest. Then am I able to pray in the pattern, as suggested further above, for God to bring healing. I also need to be open to hearing truths that can undo lies—lies I believe give the tree dark power to make sin flourish.

In my experience, there are occasions when I've felt nothing healthy or good when I know I should in some situations. This means that I was numb inside, stuck emotionally, and had unprocessed baggage to deal with. I have found that feeling the numbness within, and using the same strategies in the last paragraph works well too.

4.2: Potent Scriptures:

I used to feel that the dead structure within me was like a hidden, dark, complex vine that was wildly knotted and a nebulous mess to untie; I thought it was difficult to understand and so confusing that it disheartened and intimidated me to not even try to untangle the mess. I now have a strategy to fight the strongholds within me with Jesus' grace and truth. This strategy is built up from the following Scriptures:

1. I will never leave you nor forsake you. (Joshua 1:5)

2. Dear children, keep yourselves from idols. (1 John 5:21)

3. You will seek me and find me when you seek me with all your heart. (Jeremiah 29:13)

4. Pray unceasingly. (1 Thessalonians 5:16-18)

5. Humble yourself therefore under the mighty hand of God, that He might lift you up in due time. (1 Peter 5:6)

6. If we confess our sins, he is faithful and just, and will forgive us our sins and purify us from all unrighteousness. (1 John 1:9)

7. Repent for the Kingdom of Heaven has come near. (Mark 3:2)

8. Make restitution. (Cf. Exodus 22:1, 3-6, 14)

9. Love does no harm to a neighbor. (Romans 13:10)

10. Have faith that you have already received whatever you pray for, and it will be yours. (Mark 11:24)

11. Here I am! I stand at the door and knock. If anyone hears my voice and opens the door, I will come in and eat with that person, and they with me. (Rev. 3:20)

12. Cease striving and know that I am God. (Psalm 46:10)

13. Do not conform to the pattern of this world, but be transformed by the renewing of your mind. Then you will be able to test and approve what God's will is—his good, pleasing and perfect will. (Romans 12:2)

14. I can do all things through Him who gives me strength. (Philippians 4:13)

15. No weapon forged against you will prevail. (Isaiah 54:17)

16. Judge not and condemn not. (Cf. Luke 6:37)

17. Submit yourselves, then, to God. Resist the devil, and he will flee from you. (James 4:7)

18. Do unto others as you want them to do to you. (Matthew 7:12, aka the Golden Rule)

19. Love your neighbor as yourself. (Mark 12:31)

20. Forgive and you will be forgiven. (Luke 6:37)

21. We are not under law, but grace. (Romans 6:14)

22. Whoever believes in me, as Scripture has said, rivers of living water will flow from within them. (John 7:38)

23. For we live by faith not sight. (1 Corinthians 5:7)

24. You do not have because you do not ask God. (James 4:2)

Again, I believe that all necessary revelations that bring freedom will come gradually. Rushing and generalizing things is bad; seeking to listen to the Holy Spirit, resting in His peace, and not striving to make things happen is wisest.

Humility (being teachable) is key to making these Scriptures work in your life. Praying just any prayer modeled in this book before one: understands the vices spoken about, can remember having committed them, or knows one has such attitudes (contextually in oneself), is not wise. Always connecting with my feelings, my hunger and my thirst for right relationship with God and others when praying about them to God is wise. In doing so I am connecting my mind to my heart.

Being in touch with my feelings will put me in touch with my thinking. I can then renew my thinking as I continue to seek God with all my heart. I will eventually find God and the freedom He offers in the process. Being connected to the source of my feelings, such as unhealthy desires, anger, faulty beliefs, poor thinking, bad commitments, and misguided loyalties means I can repent from them more fully with Jesus' help and grace. Disconnection often means I have stuffed away, denied, compartmentalized, or become blind to the nature of my attitudes and their vices.

I will now make some important definitions (along with some commentary) that have made the dismantling process easier, understandable, and possible for me to work through. These working definitions are what this book hinges on; without them the contents of this book are meaningless and have no power. Biblical language and concepts can often have skeptical, religious ideas superimposed on them or negative, worldly connotations, and so they lose their meaning and power. Who uses the word "repent" in public these days? It is often misunderstood by people both outside and inside the church. These definitions below are meant to put us on the same page and move us forward.

4.3: Working Definitions

Ceaselessly Pray:

To ceaselessly pray means to replace our constant monologue in our head with two-way dialogue with God.

This is done by reasoning with God through faith. And letting His wisdom and life spontaneously flow like a river, into the otherwise stagnant pool of our minds and hearts, to bring life, joy, relationship, and renewal. It also means to express our feelings honestly to God so we can honestly process them. The Holy Spirit gives us wisdom on how to make wise decisions that are non-judgmental and kind in nature so our relationships grow and don't stagnate.

For a long time, and because of a half-truth, I saw God as a power to be used, accessed, and worshipped for my benefit alone. I was in error. God deserves our worship for his glory—not mine. God also needs to be respected, cared for, and loved just like we as humans seek after such things for ourselves—after all, we are made in His image. He also seeks to be valued, cherished, and seen as important for His own sake because He is three persons (Father, Son, and Holy Spirit) with likes and dislikes. He seeks to be in healthy relationships just like we do.

To the degree that we fear breaking God's heart and desire to respect Him as someone who wants to be loved, this is the degree we will supernaturally regard (love) others too. God became man, and in doing so He chose to become dependent on our love, which ultimately comes from Him. So, seeking God to manipulate Him into giving us what we want is unhealthy. Seeking to give and receive from God is healthier than taking from Him and using Him. Asking the Holy Spirit a question and listening for an answer can be very straight forward when we know the promises and principles found in the Scriptures and believe them.

When we come into God's presence we shouldn't do so lightheartedly. Otherwise, we won't take God's answers seriously, and we won't be as discerning concerning God's voice. "We can test the source of the communications we hear (after having asked a question to the Holy Spirit) by simply asking the source, "Is this the 'flesh' or the Spirit speaking?" If it is the "flesh" then reject the message; if it is the Spirit then we can further test the content until we are sure the Holy Spirit has spoken to us."[19]

Mark Virkler's book on two-way prayer through journaling called *4 Keys to Hearing God's Voice* is also very helpful. The keys are meant to give structure to the process of journaling and they are based on the Bible. They help one to listen, remember, and reflect on what actually is said by God in a non-judgmental and less skeptical fashion. He provides biblical tests to discern what

---

[19] Paraphrase from Brad Jersak's eBook: *Can You Hear Me?* from Chapter 4 called, "Was That Just My Imagination?" used with permission.

is written, and is well worth the read and practice.

Both books have been foundational to arriving at the contents found in this book.

Some prayers unleash great power, grace and peace by dismantling sin strongholds and bring in virtues to replace our sins. Other prayers (even said in faith and humility) can seem unanswered. We should not doubt or fall into unbelief about such prayers. We walk by faith. God uses all healthy prayers if not in the present then in the future. Walking by faith and believing God has our backs helps the answers to these quiet prayers take on substance in our relating with others as well as with God. The moment we fall into unbelief in an area, then the devil robs us of God's gift. When we walk by faith believing God's promises, then they have a chance of materializing, maybe not overnight but gradually.

Attitudes:

Attitudes are commitments to beliefs we make about objects, ideas, events, or other people. Attitudes can be neutral, positive, or negative. Conscious attitudes are beliefs that guide our decisions and behaviors. Unconscious attitudes are beliefs that also influence our decisions and behavior.

Thoughts and ideas trigger feelings. Whereas beliefs about who we are or what we or others deserve, determine our attitudes. In changing our thoughts, we change our feelings. In changing our beliefs, we change our attitudes. Feelings come and go whereas attitudes have so much more staying power for good and evil. Attitudes are energies (commitments to behaviors) that have likes, dislikes, and desires that can carry judgments that determine some of our emotions and behaviors. In getting rid of bad attitudes we no longer want, we need to give up the lies believed, and judgments associated with them, and the energy (commitment) that translates into the behaviors. Renewing the mind and heart through confession, together with repenting in prayer, forgiving people, and seeking God's will, is often the way to do just that.

I realized early on that my thoughts, beliefs and attitudes create feelings and emotions. And I also later realized that I was in the habit of believing my thoughts, beliefs and attitudes because the emotions they created were so strong and real. They often made me feel very weak, powerless and frantic for relief. And I saw no way out of this for a long time except to change my different thoughts, beliefs, and attitudes that materialized each time in different contexts. This seemed more easily said than done. At times it seemed overwhelming. Then it occurred to me that I could confess this dynamic (i.e. believing certain stuff because my emotions were so strong and real) to Jesus as unhealthy, i.e. sinful, and give it up with Jesus' help through faith through grace and truth. This freed me from giving my feelings and emotions so much power.

So, there are times when changing my thoughts, beliefs and attitudes is a must. But not always. Sometimes confessing to God this dynamic mess and taking back the power I've given to my feelings and emotions to determine reality clears the way to becoming sane again with both legs planted solidly in the earth.

Renewing Our Mind and Heart:

Renewing our mind and heart involves confession (which is a must), repentance from sin and sin strongholds in prayer, giving up fears, forgiving people, and giving up judgments. Then we reprogram the mind's pathways and the heart's habits. Below are some helpful strategies you can use to achieve complete renewal in problem areas. In reprogramming pathways and habits in the mind and heart, as "the tree of knowledge of good and evil" is dismantled and removed, we deal more frequently with the "sin nature":

1. Whenever we encounter an ugly attitude (like "self-pity" for example) that is triggered in some way, then the first thing to do is confess it to God and ask Him to heal our minds from it. Self-pity means we are indulging in weakness. Giving up feeling sorry for oneself and choosing to be strong instead is the path to take.

This is easier said than done when self-pity is a stronghold, but here is an example of how God led me to repent from a stronghold of self-pity. It has the following Sin-Conduit Structure:

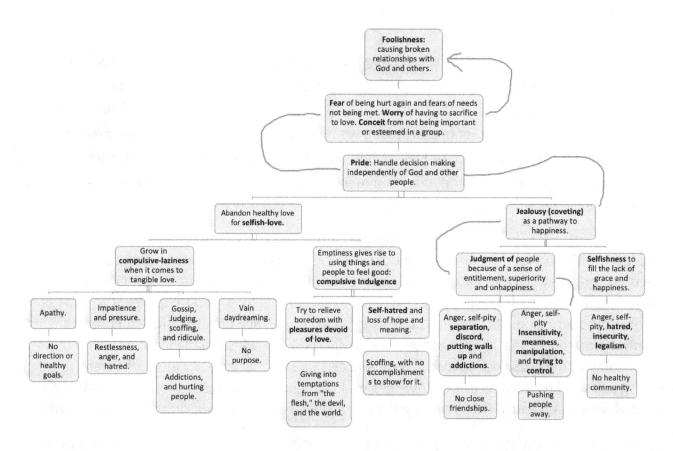

After the Sin-Conduit Structure above, we get the Sin-Anatomy Table below:

Self-pity	Judging	Coveting & Jealousy	Pride	Fear, Worry, & Conceit	Foolishness
	<=	<=	<=	<=	<= Cause and Effect
Out of self-pity I try to argue or manipulate people so they like me, respect me, or become friendly.	Furious that people don't brighten up. Furious that they don't endorse or congratulate me on my efforts to please them.	Covet respect... but it eludes me. So I feel frustrated, violated.	It all lands on me and my shoulders. I am the center of the universe. So I will pretend to do what is strong.	Feel lost, and abandoned and I worry that no one cares about me.	Weak approach: I don't know what to do.
Want to implode and cry poor me because of an unfair audience and world....					
Confession & Repenting in Faith =>	=>	=>	=>	=>	

Prayer:

Lord Jesus, I confess that I'm sorely tempted out of self-pity to manipulate people into liking me, respecting me, and honoring me. I admit my anger is behind this self-pity because people seem to treat me like the weak person I feel like I am at times. I admit that I feel frustrated by the lack of respect I seem to get and covet. I feel this is all on my shoulders, and out of pride I pretend to be unconvincingly strong. This comes from the feeling of being lost and abandoned and believing the lie that no one else cares about my situation. This comes from my weak approach that says, "I don't know what to do," in so many situations that ask for confidence and assertiveness.

I give up saying "no" to this, with your help Jesus. Lord God, I regret all this sinful weakness and ask for your forgiveness, and I choose to give it all up with your help in faith instead. I choose to walk by faith, doing what I believe I should do instead of being paralyzed by the belief that I don't know what to do. Thank you Jesus for loving me. Amen!

2. When it comes to self-pity ask yourself if you want to be negative or positive? Realize that negativity draws negative stuff to you. Realize that positivity draws positive stuff to you. Self-pity is negative in nature. So choose positive attitudes instead of self-pity. Put another way, choose to act like an adult (mature) and not like a child (immature)

in the face of seemingly negative challenges. We don't passively wait around for this; instead we do it with God's grace either by choosing to be mature directly or if this doesn't work, then by asking the Holy Spirit to heal our minds and trusting in expectant faith that He will. God is faithful.

3. Replace believing in lies with believing in practical, commonsense truths: those found in the Bible, those that God inserts into your mind spontaneously, or those through conversations with everyday people.

4. Welcome Jesus' presence and become teachable by incorporating His truth, teaching, promises, and grace into the different contexts in your personal and relational life.

5. Sometimes, you can be so engaged in mentally saying "no" to a bad attitude without success, that the healthiest thing one can do is to pray: "Jesus with your help I give up saying 'no' to the bad attitude," and "Jesus I give up the bad attitude with your help in faith." I have done this and found tangible success in areas that had stymied me for years. The reason this strategy works is because it moves me from "self-righteously attempting to save myself through my own will power" to inviting "God into the repentance process through His grace." Sometimes the greatest obstacles to freedom are self-effort, anger, and self-pity. Sometimes the "no" we use on ourselves can be so self-loathing, mean, pressure driven, desperate, and utterly without faith in God's offer to help bring closure—no wonder it gives no success. Praying like this in the areas that trigger: desires for skewed justice, vengeance, brutality, hatred, and self-mutilation really will be a game changer.

   I have done this and found tangible success.

6. Ask God regularly to replace the unwanted vices in us with the gifts of opposite virtues: if we struggle with compulsive-indulging, we ask Him for self-control; If we struggle with conceit, we ask for the ability to respect all people along with ourselves; if we struggle with pride, we ask for humility; If we struggle with selfishness, we ask for generosity; If we struggle with cowardice we ask for courage; If we struggle with judging we ask for tolerance; etc. But we have to ask God in faith and not with double mindedness to receive His gifts.

7. Both anger and self-pity can be used to pressure, force, or manipulate change in any realm when they are inspired by the "sin nature." But sometimes self-pity can be so intense that it hides the fact that we are using anger for selfish motives too. If we are using anger, then self-pity often accompanies it too. We ought to examine both possibilities when we are struggling and want freedom from our compulsions.

   When the "sin nature" is active by way of using anger or self-pity to get my way, I have learned that I need to say, "I accept you, but I don't need you right now." This has to be said directly to the "sin nature" (attitudes) when they are initiated or triggered. If I try to say no to them, I just give them more power and that means I need to expend more energy and time to wrestle with or resist them. I need to pray,

"I give it up, with your help Jesus, through faith." I have learned that I need to accept my "sin nature" and not leave it out of my calculations.

8. Take advantage of this strategy: "Event + Reaction = Outcome." This means that between an *event* and the *outcome* is a span of time where we can reprogram our mind and heart settings (*reaction*) instead of having the old unwanted junk codes to repeat continually. For instance, if we are angry with ourselves for falling into a sin and are inclined to use angry pressure to change it, then we can say in speaking to the anger "I accept you but don't need you right now"; praying, "I give it up, with your help Jesus, through faith"; and saying to Jesus, "Your grace is sufficient." And then we ask ourselves: "What do I want most instead of this old sin habit?" We then decide on an answer and prayerfully commit to thinking and reacting in ways that make the most of every opportunity instead of participating in a sin habit. Gradually a new habit pattern replaces the old habit pattern and we are free in the problem area. The way I look at it is that I am going to be stoked one way or another when people cause things to happen that I become aware of. And the emotions and attitudes welded to such felt events can seem so hopelessly determined when they are not grace based. But I get to choose how I'm going to react after any event has been felt by me. We don't have to change or agree with an event, try to suppress our feelings surrounding it, or feel hopelessly enslaved to an unkind attitude attached to it after the fact. I can replace negative reactions with positive, kind, caring, peaceful, and compassionate reactions when the strongholds are gone.

9. If we use self-pity and anger inappropriately (and they have been *big* issues in our lives) then going back in our memories and processing them in prayer, from the past up to the present, will bring healing and joy. One root of self-pity is being selfish. To rid myself of most of my self-pity I need to dismantle all the Sin-Conduit Structures that contain selfishness in my personal "tree of knowledge of good and evil." This is done through strategic prayer, strategic truth, giving up my commitments to always being first or being in love with myself, and making new commitments to loving God and the people in my life. This works when self-pity is a result of selfishness. But self-pity can also be harnessed by my "sin nature" to get my way and grow "the tree of knowledge of good and evil" within me. Self-pity, when it rears its ugly head, needs to be diagnosed and treated accordingly.

10. We can accuse God of being unfair consciously, and we can even believe it subconsciously somewhere in our makeup, and so we pout a lot and get full of self-pity and negativity because of it. To stop going to these places of unfairness (a second source of self-pity) in our minds every time something goes wrong, we need to give up pointing our finger at God. We do this in prayer by confessing and repenting our judgment of God as unfair. And then we practice getting in touch with our gratitude, and we focus on positively loving the people in our lives with God's help. Remember, life can be unfair, but God is *love*.

11. Remaining committed to a view that God is unfair leads to self-pity, jealousy, demanding things, and using anger to get our way. Choosing to see life through the eyes of grace instead of a cup that is half-empty, leads to making the most of every opportunity. This is done one situation at a time. If we pour all our energy into being happy, then happiness will elude us. We can't work up the emotional state of happiness, but we can choose to be grateful in all our circumstances because God is good. Grace leads to joy. Gratitude and praise directed at God are key to silencing a lot of self-pity, but it must be done wisely without shoving issues under carpets. The choice is ours.

12. Don't attempt to do everything by yourself. Let God into the picture because He cares for you deeply. We are not alone or abandoned—Jesus is with us to help. He will never leave us nor forsake us. We shouldn't think we are by ourselves. We need to remind ourselves often that we aren't orphans. When connected to Jesus there is peace; with peace the attraction to sin or compulsive-indulging is lessened, and so we practice self-control more victoriously. This is a result of grace and God's empowering presence.

13. Often we set our hearts on opportunities in the past that never worked out for us but that we thought would make us happy. We need to consult God about these disappointments and give up those past longings for happiness that make us irritable, negative, and self-pitying. And then choose new commitments like loving God fully and others as ourselves instead.

14. Get in touch with the joy of God's salvation in your life. Joy, when we have it, oils the squeaky wheel of annoyances: it moves us away from being petty, anal, judgmental, and quick tempered; it aids us in our attempts to love and handle life maturely; it stops the cycle of self-pity.

Confession

I use the word "confess" a lot in this book. To make a confession we do the following: admit contritely, gently, accurately and genuinely our sins (our unhealthy attitudes, their story, and their history to God); agree with God that they are wrong, and say we are sorry for them (regret having committed them); request to be forgiven them and healed of them by God. When we do this, 1 John 1:9 promises God will forgive us and cleanse us from all unrighteousness. We need to claim this promise during confession, after confession, and as we seek to repent, because if we don't then there is little chance of cleansing and healing coming from God. Sometimes the key that breaks the power of a sin habit comes quickly, other times we need to be patient. We ought to not give up.

It is very important for us to not just intellectualize confession. We need to connect with our emotions, and that means getting in touch with the peace that comes from being forgiven by

God. We need to experience the joy, stability, divine touch, and breath of life that confession and forgiveness brings into our lives through the Holy Spirit.

While confessing my sins to God, I have learned that it is a bad idea to always speak in generalities. When we can put more meat than bones into our prayers we should do so. Lies have a better chance of being exposed when we get specific and look at the details more closely. We need to try to understand the unhealthy energy, attitudes, and mechanisms working in our heart and mind when it comes to sin. When we do this, the Holy Spirit can speak truth into the different areas of our lives and set us free.

Before attempting to repent from a sin, one needs to first confess one's sin in the problem area to God.

When we hold onto promises from God we are walking in faith. In the same way, when I get a promise fulfilled like being cleansed after confession, then I will know automatically who fulfilled it, and will continue to walk in faith with thanksgiving. God gives to us because He loves us, and not because we have muscles of faith. Faith is like a door that opens to let God's provision in. God loves us even when we don't have faith, and gives to all people (both good and bad) because He cares for us all. God loved us while we were still His enemy.

Grace

Grace is God's unconditional love for us, as well as His empowering presence. Unconditional love means we are loved whether we do good, do bad or are apathetic. This means God does not love us less when we do bad, nor do we have to earn His love by doing good works. Grace, as far as God's empowering presence is concerned, comes through a humble faith and trust in Jesus: that He has not left us as orphans, that He cares for us, and that He helps us fight our battles. For me, I invite grace by asking Jesus for it, and believe I have received it with thanksgiving. I choose to live like I have that grace.

On the other hand, judging and pride swallow up grace, so repenting of such sin strongholds is critical for God's grace and presence to be felt in my life. When I don't feel grace I still trust that it is there, because Jesus promised that He would never leave nor forsake us.[20]

Repenting in Prayer From a Sin

The word "repent" means to renew or change our minds about our sin and the lies we believed that made us give into the temptations. And this is always done with God's help in prayer.

---

[20] Cf. Deuteronomy 31:8

Practically, this means praying something like:

> "Dear God, I give up saying "no," in my own self-righteous energy, to the sin of
> "_____." And in faith, with your help and grace Lord Jesus, I give up the sin instead. I
> ask you to help me renew my mind, by showing me the lies I believed that caused me to
> sin so I can give them up."

Carefully search your mind and memory, and ask the Holy Spirit to speak spontaneously to you—to tell you the lies you believed. List them and then give them up one at a time with God's help, by praying:

> "Lord God, I give up believing the following lies: "_____," with your help."

Note, the flesh or "sin nature" might insert misleading information so one will need to sift through what comes up.

Next, seek contextual truths—common sense wisdom that grounds the renewal process deep in the heart. We must believe truth with the heart as well as with the mind so the lies don't have the same power anymore. Then ask God to replace the vices with the opposite virtues, which are God's gifts. Claim the grace granted to us in Jesus, through faith, that enables us to live victoriously. Choose to live mindful that grace and truth is being imparted to us, and be dependent on Jesus, who won't abandon us.

Finally, make restitution and apologize where needed. Do no harm to both those you need to apologize to and those you need to make restitution to.[21]

The sin should be dealt a blow, but often there can be many roots depending on the history involved, the energy flow in the sin tree structure, and the dynamics involved. Each root or branch needs to be dealt with for the past to be resolved.

This book gives a systematic way to uncover the lies and fears that make certain strongholds in our lives, along with a strategy to dismantle the same strongholds. To do this we need to deal with our sinful attitudes in prayer.

Repenting in Prayer From Sinful Attitudes

An approach to "repenting in prayer" that works for me is outlined here. You need to be as specific as possible, while being humble and contrite, so you can get to the roots of each matter and not sloppily sweep things under carpets.

For instance, just praying, "Lord God, I repent in faith with your help from my pride," does not

---

[21] Cf. Exodus 22:1, 3-6, 14, and Romans 13:10

by itself get to the roots of any matter. Since prayer has to do with being honest, which can be painful at times, developing a personal language that relates to your faith relationship with God is very important when it comes to forgiveness and healing.

Generally speaking the prayers in this book (as a guideline) are composed in this manner:

I can use the following prayer if I am dealing with any one of the following attitudes: self-pity, demandingness, fear, pride, superiority, arrogance, conceit, selfish-love, being uncaring, envy, inferiority, coveting, selfishness, jealousy, judging, resentment, anger, hatred, greed, legalism, sloth (compulsive-laziness), compulsive-indulging, emptiness, being anal, being petty, being a jerk etc.:

> "Dear God, I give up saying 'no' self-righteously to the sin attitude of '_____' and give it up instead with your help in faith. And I give up, with your help in faith, being committed to and believing: '_____'."

For pride I might say:

> "I'm the center of the universe"; "I am most important"; "Others need to come last"; or "I'm better than them."

For judging I might say:

> "I'm good and they are bad."
>
> "There is always an asshole in the crowd."
>
> "Beggars can't be choosers."
>
> "I'm intelligent and they are stupid."
>
> "They deserve my scorn, mockery, laughter, wrath, disdain, judging, aggravation, impatience, pettiness, lack of charity etc."
>
> "I deserve fairness more than they do."

For coveting I might say:

> "My concerns are more important than those belonging to other people etc."

Then I'd continue to pray:

> "When I did or said '_____' while relating to the person '_____', and I'm sorry for wanting to (or actually) hurting these people to protect my self-image or protect myself against threats or possible hurts. I therefore ask you, the Holy Spirit, to replace these sins in my life with their corresponding opposite virtues '_____' as your gifts to me. I choose to submit my tongue, eyes, ears, mind, body, energy, mechanics, money, possessions, influence, desires, beliefs and will, to you the Living God: in your energy and leading,

through faith in Jesus, to be used for love and not in the service of the sins I have just confessed here.

Next, I'd make restitution and apologize where needed. Doing no harm to both those I need to make restitution to and those I need to apologize to.[22]

"I choose to humble myself, seeking to healthily love you God and the people I meet, with your grace and truth Lord Jesus. And to not pretend that I'm healthier than what I am. And I ask you the Living God to heal me, as I accept you Jesus as my Lord, Truth, Savior, Healer, Grace, Peace and Life Giver—the one I'm dependent on."

Later, when renewing the mind, I will want to counter the sin or lie (i.e. for pride) with something like:

"God is the center of the universe."

"I want to love others like I want to be loved"

"I don't see all things clearly."

"I choose to become teachable with God's help."

"I choose to care for people with God's help."

"I choose to be kind to people with God's help."

"I am God's workmanship wired to be compassionate, caring and giving."

"I am the light of the world like Jesus said and I choose to live this out daily."

"I am the salt of the earth like Jesus said and I choose to live this out daily."

"I am hardwired by God to be patient with people; I therefore choose to be patient with people."

And for other sins I adopt biblical or common sense truths that will help to set me free to love.

If, like me, you carry such baggage, then you will want to give up, with Jesus' help, the following motives: unhealthily protecting the identity or self-esteem thinking "I am better than others"; expecting and demanding from others that I be first; trying to control people; expecting others to live foremost according to my values or morality; coveting power, wealth, or sex; "I got to get what they have" thinking; "it's all about me" thinking; "I can't do it" thinking; demanding, grasping, or having an active sense of entitlement; "I got to get even" thinking; despising something about a person or a group of people; hating a person, active superiority or racism; pressure or manipulation; selling out or betrayal; expectations of perfectionism; or other

---

[22] Cf. Exodus 22:1, 3-6, 14, and Romans 13:10

misguided ideals etc.

And, if you carry such baggage, you will want to give up with Jesus' help anyone of the following commitments: making rash vows, wearing masks, seeking revenge, getting even, lashing out, scoffing, cynicism, pouting, negativity, contempt, judging, letting walls go up and pushing people away, projecting arrogance, uncontrolled anger, hostility, insensitivity, verbal abuse, meanness, exerting force or violence, pressuring or manipulating, lying, stealing, hurting others, not taking "no" for an answer, violating boundaries, acting like a jerk, making waves and demands to get one's way at all costs, communicating an "I'm better or intelligent," vs. "They're bad, worse, stupid," mindset etc.

For decades, I tried to motivate inner change, repentance, self-control, and people who annoyed me, with my anger. This needs to be abandoned because human anger has nothing to do with the righteousness of God and is a strategy that does not work. The good thing is we can become aware of such anger in the different contexts of our lives (including our histories) and both give it up and replace it with gentleness and trust instead, with Jesus' help in prayer. Realizing anger as a means to change does not work, and instead using healthy, gentle thinking and motivations, is life changing. Being hard on oneself because of temptation, while sinning, or after sinning is not healthy. This needs to be prayed through so the love of God motivates us instead.

It is crucial to invite, depend on, and believe Jesus for His grace as one tackles life. God has not left us as orphans. He is with us. To celebrate grace (God's empowering presence) just as much as welcoming truth to build up our interior and relational lives is the clincher to being able to live free from the above negative strongholds. We do this by practicing repentance and abiding in Jesus as the Spirit leads.

Giving up Fear

To continue the act of repentance we need to drive out our fears (insecurities and instabilities) completely and allow God's love to flow into us and out of us to others. This requires that the grace of God be poured into and applied to our lives. This is done best through friendship with God via "Journaling Prayer" which is the two-way prayer as described and practiced by Mark Virkler.

We all hunger for God. When we spend time with Him through journaling, and allow His words to penetrate and enter the otherwise stagnant pools of our lives, then His grace accompanies the truth He speaks and we are set free to love. We are healed of the toxic streams of energy and bad habits, also known as "strongholds" in this book.

We can pray about fears like we do with bad attitudes, but fears often carry a lot more baggage. Giving up or repenting of fears more thoroughly is a little different, because we are often aware of our fears. Naming them helps us to see what is giving them power in our lives. Here is a way to deal with unreasonable fears in prayer more thoroughly:

Step 1. Talk to God about where you are at, and let Him speak to you through the thoughts in your head.

Step 2. Ask yourself, and ask God which of the fears that you struggle with are unreasonable. Write down each fear (i.e. intimacy, being made a fool of, being hurt, losing, going home empty, being written off, being "put in a box," that you won't have what others have, that you will not have friends, being left out or left behind, being ridiculed or laughed at, not being acknowledged, not being valued, not being cared about etc.).

Step 3. For each fear ask yourself, and the Holy Spirit what lies you are believing behind each fear. Write them down. (i.e. believing you're completely bad or you can't do it; going by what if they do "such and such" negative thing to you; thinking there isn't enough for everyone—that some might go without, so you have to do everything moral or immoral to get your deserved share; reasoning you've got to use people at all costs to get your way no matter how humiliating it is for them etc.).

This all leads to darkness, not living in the moment, and not accepting people where they are at. The possibility of saying yes is found in Jesus. We must have faith: in God, in people, and in ourselves. Otherwise we draw negativity to ourselves and live without hope: sowing negativity and reaping negativity. Grace is the most powerful thing in relationships when invited in, because it believes the best about people, and treats them in the healthiest ways possible.

Step 4. Write down the sins you act out when you entertain each fear and lie you wrote down. (i.e. worrying, pretending or acting like someone we are not, despairing, lying, eating, manipulating, trying to control people or their opinions, cheating, being mean, acting like a jerk, playing it safe, not taking chances... etc.)

Step 5. Along with the sins write down the reactions to the fears (i.e. embarrassment, falling for catch-22's, using faulty thinking, seeking power out of pride, showing up way too early or too late etc.).

Step 6. Then for each fear, lie, sin and reaction combination pray something like the following:

"Lord Jesus, with your help through faith in you, I give up self-righteously saying 'no' to the fears, lies, sins, and reactions mentioned, and instead I give up the sin of "_____" (Step 4) and related reactions "_____" (Step 5) because they are wrong. I give up believing the lies of "_____" (Step 3) that helped enslave me to the sin of indulging in the unreasonable fears of "_____" (Step 2). I give up this fear with your help and I choose to believe your truth. I embrace the promises found in the Bible, especially the promises of "_____" (i.e. peace, grace, mercy, perfect love that casts out all fear, relationship with God through Jesus, Living Waters, never being forsaken, courage, bravery, having my needs looked after etc.). Lord Jesus, I receive your forgiveness for all my sins along with the fulfillment of all these promises in my life that I ask for. I receive this all intellectually, emotionally, and as your beloved child. There may be no hurts, just lies I foolishly believed that inspire my fears, but if there are hurts, then I further pray: I choose to forgive "_____" (people who hurt me in a way that helps trigger my fears).

I choose to stand in your grace, to love people, and to now resist the devil and his efforts to nullify the graces given me through you Jesus. And I ask you Jesus to help me renew my thoughts and beliefs with common sense truth, and the wisdom found in the Scriptures (make up your mind to search for it, ask people what they think, and ask God what He thinks; imagine what it looks like and choose to commit to living out the virtues along with bravery through the rich graces Jesus pours into our lives). Almighty God, thank you for setting me free from these sins and from indulging in the fears above. I pray this in Jesus' name. Amen.

Fear is so powerful that it can swallow up the caring and compassion we want to show others. The Lord made me aware that I had two fears that led to selfishness that stole the compassion that God put into my heart. They were:

1. Fear of not getting things done because of inflexibility, and

2. Fear of falling behind on "to-do" lists at work and at home because of inflexibility.

These fears found their way into many nooks and crannies in my life. When I prayed as suggested above, I became free of these fears. I became more in touch with my compassionate nature. I no longer froze, or panicked or went to places of selfishness when I was called upon to go out of my way. I grew in maturity. I began to struggle much less with self-pity in this context.

Another fear the Lord led me to give up was: "Fear that I don't have enough time" when people made requests from me. This fear led to much anxiety, guilt and compulsive laziness in my life. It led me to live for an empty future. It made me more selfish, and less able to enjoy the moments in the present.

Often fears are triggered by the unknown, by threats, by trauma, and by hurt. The above suggested prayer can deal with such. Over time we can accumulate many strongholds of fear in our minds and spirits that can, through pride, trigger all the unwanted strongholds spoken about in this book. These fears can be completely vanquished through the suggested prayer above in the context of a love relationship with God. Two-way journaling prayer—in this context—doesn't mean we necessarily focus on the topics of fear, insecurity, and instability all the time, but it is a good idea to visit when the Spirit leads. Journaling is broader than just talking about fear or sin all the time. We give God the freedom to direct the conversation as He pleases, and we can ask Him whatever we want that interests us, because He is kind, gentle, warm, loving, gracious, and compassionate.

Prayer Example

"Lord Jesus, I give up my self-righteous 'no's' to the fears of intimacy and of being hurt, and I instead give up these fears with your help. I choose to give up my cowardice, protectionism, cold rigidness, not wanting to be honest, deceptiveness, and my hiding from people because of my pride. I give up being prideful, putting up walls, and creating distance from people. I confess these as wrong and ask for your forgiveness and healing. I receive these gifts emotionally and intellectually through faith from you the Living God. I also forgive my first girlfriend for not respecting me as a person with feelings, dignity, and flaws; and I forgive myself for the way I let her hurt me. I choose to love those who cross my path and I accept the pain that accompanies doing so. I ask for the gift of intimacy, courage, and strength to be myself. Jesus, thank you for your grace, never leaving my side, and sustaining your peace within me by your presence. Amen.

The strategy to confront negative strongholds is to admit they are in our lives and to say to them that we don't need them right now, because God provides for our needs with His grace, truth, and peace. All sins are a result of falsely believing that they will fulfill our needs or save us somehow; the key to moving on is admitting this in each context, mourning the losses incurred (because the devil's promises amount to emptiness in the end), and committing to and connecting with Jesus as Prince of Peace.

We need to do this emotionally as well as intellectually. In this way, we count previous strongholds of sin dead, and embrace the full life promised by Jesus. Nature hates vacuums so we should replace sin with virtues. Virtues come from clean energy (grace), peace, the presence of God along with healthy truth. The presence of God is the Holy Spirit, we need to ask Him to overcome our sins.

Some attitudes can have many layers or many roots and we need to be patient until each layer or all roots are eventually dismantled.

Masks and "the tree of knowledge of good and evil" go together. Adam and Eve put on masks after they ate from this tree; they felt shame and immediately had fears so they tried to protect themselves with leaf coverings after their innocence was stolen. God knew that would not work, so He chose to shed blood to give them leather skin coverings to help remove their shame and fears. This shedding is prophetic of Jesus' blood being spilt so that our masks (idols of fear protection) could also be washed away leaving us pure, clean, and able to enjoy rich community once again.

There is fear of being shamed, and then there is fear of people; they aren't always the same. Both need to be dealt with in prayer and renewing one's mind with the promises of grace and truth found in Scripture.

The process of repenting prayer asks us to deal with the lies we believed in the moments we were seduced to become slaves of certain sins that became strongholds in our lives. These lies are the reasons why we use certain idols to try to wrongly satisfy our needs.

For instance, if we were hurt by being rejected, we can be deceived into believing the lie that through a conceited attitude we will protect our self-images and maintain a sense that we are still likable. Or we can come to think that compulsive-laziness is the answer to having peace in our hearts. Or we can be deceived into thinking that food will give us peace. These idols don't satisfy us, can be very expensive, and besides marring our personalities and bodies confuse us about our identities.

The above prayers and strategies are ways of committing to a clean conscience with the help of God; committing to renewing the mind, attitudes, expectations, thinking, and beliefs we have through grace, in a way that changes our actions from sin to love through gentle obedience to Jesus as Lord and Savior.

For instance, if we were rejected as young children (like I was), we could vow to aim hatred and malice at those who rejected us because of the hurt, and we may find that vow still operative towards those who later in life seemingly threaten our self-image, identity and sense of safety. This can go very deep and be unhealthily layered in our hearts with meanness, scoffing, scorn, judging, "us = good" vs. "them = bad" thinking, contempt, negativity, and insensitivity pouring out of us at others when triggered (like I did). But just as sadly and importantly we must realize that this meanness, scoffing, scorn, judging, negativity, and being hard on people can also be directed at ourselves for letting the first and subsequent rejections to happen. We need to forgive both the agents of our hurts and ourselves. And we need to give up our judgments and attacks against God for letting the hurt happen in the first place.

Further, we could believe the lie (like I did) that we will be better than others through self-effort, vow to be perfect always, and eventually come to believe the lie that we are better than others. This can become so habitually ingrained within us, distorting and defiling our personalities and self-image if not reversed. I have found countering such streams of prideful energy with targeted truth to be very helpful.

I have found that when such a wound goes very deep, situations that challenge my self-image will trigger the sins mentioned in this context towards others, and these sins need to be confessed and repented from in prayer (also dealing with pride, fear, and negativity in this context) and confronted with strategic truth each time they materialize to get rid of the streams of bad energy. But part of the cancer is the hatred directed towards oneself within, which also needs to be confessed and repented from in genuine prayer. If we hate ourselves, then we will hate others.

Our words have power for good or bad and using them for good can bring freedom. Sin is no longer our master when Jesus sets us free by His grace and truth flowing through us. This is done gradually area after area with our cooperation. To successfully put to death the sinful attitude we need a clean energy in our prayers, tone of speech, beliefs, thinking, will and efforts.

And to also say yes to the corresponding virtuous acts, in obedience to Jesus, made possible by grace and truth. When we use clean energy we will see great victories in our emotional life and attitudes. It only takes a little leaven to raise a whole batch of dough. We can't throw out negative energy with negative energy. We all have safe places within us, no matter how sinful we are, where together with faith in Jesus, we can conquer the darkness within with His light and grace.

Occasionally, we will react with a carnal attitude, and this should inspire confessing and repenting in prayer. But sometimes the emotions of the attitude linger, and we may try to wrestle with it. This latter is counterproductive. Confessing and repenting give the emotion or attitude less power; whereas wrestling with it does not. The more one focuses on a negative attitude and tries to wrestle with it the more power one gives to it. God says, "Not by human might, but by my power." God's power works with truth and sets us free.

After dealing with visible sins, vices (pride, using people, coveting, selfishness etc.) and fears thoroughly through prayer, the next step is to deal with broken relationships. This can mean having to forgive the people who hurt us contextually.

Sometimes I've prayed, as suggested in this book, but it did not bring complete freedom in an area. When this happens then I know that I have to go deeper in prayer, and I'm usually missing one or more truths needed to push the devil more completely out of that troublesome area.

Forgiveness

When we choose to forgive somebody, we are jettisoning our bad energy towards the person and choosing good energy towards them instead. This is what it means to have a pure heart. We don't even have to use the words, "I forgive you," with them. We can just decide to give up the hardness, blackness, coldness, un-grace, judgment and hate in our hearts; and instead say yes to loving the person with clean energy, and refuse to bring up the past because we have forgiven them from our hearts. This is based on living out the Golden Rule together with grace. We want unconditional love (i.e. grace) so we grant the same grace to everyone. When it comes to judging someone who did us wrong this kind of forgiveness is most needed, otherwise we remain wounded. We forgive for our own sake. If we don't forgive people who piss us off, it won't necessarily affect their destiny but it will affect ours. I choose to forgive others because it is healthy for me to do so, and because I *really* want to be a good person. I can't be a good person if I cut off my love from anyone. A way to forgive is to pray something like this without minimizing what they did:

"Lord Jesus, with your help I give up my judgments towards "_____"
and I give up my conceit in this area too.
With your help in faith, I therefore now forgive: "_____"
for what they did to me when "_____."
And with your help Lord God in faith I give up my wishes for revenge against them now:
I give up the darkness and hatred in my heart,
I set both this person free and myself too,
and I choose to love them because this brings peace and happiness to me.
Thank you for healing me
and helping me to say yes to loving this person instead.

Amen."

I can't be friends with everyone. Yes, I am called to forgive everyone who sins against me, but if they are toxic, unkind, judgmental, uncaring or basically rub me the wrong way all the time, then a friendship is just not practical. I get to choose my friends; I don't have to be friends with someone just because they want it. Forgiveness yes, but friends not always.

This goes both ways. Not everyone wants to be my friend. Accepting this is very healthy. I can't hang around others hoping they will notice me and pretend they aren't ignoring my needs; this needs to be abandoned, given up in prayer, and processed so I can move on. Love does not demand to be loved by others.

When I have been hurt, Satan floods my mind with fear, lies, and judgments that are designed to form resentments. These help to grow "the tree of knowledge of good and evil" within me. Forgiving those involved, forgiving myself, and giving up judging and attacking God will invite grace, healing, peace, warmth, and caring into my heart, and help me to dismantle the tree within so love can thrive.

Moreover, sometimes it seems impossible to forgive no matter how much I wrestle with doing so. I have found that when this happens the issue is not so much that I can't forgive, but that I need to repent from my conceit. Pride blocks me from forgiving others.

It is crucial that I capture the full essence of my thinking, emotions, bad and good attitudes, sins, fears, reasoning, and resentments on paper when it comes to processing compulsions, baggage, annoyances, being unforgiving, heartache, and confusion. I must take it all to God in order for Him to give me healing through His touches, insights, truth, wisdom and grace. As I confess and repent in faith from my sins, and make adjustments to my paradigms and expectations, the "tree of knowledge of good and evil" within me will be dismantled. After I have done this, then using "I" statements to renew my thinking is the next wise thing to do.

"I" Statements

Giving up my judgments of the persons who wronged me paves the way to easily forgive them from my heart. A way of uprooting further judgments towards people who have hurt or violated me is for me to use "I" statements.

"I" statements follow the formula:

I feel "_____" when "_____" because "_____" and would like "_____."

They are to be simple, non-threatening, and non-judgmental statements, without accusations, name calling, or putdowns.

"I" statements are meant to be used after I confess and repent from judgments, resentments, hostility, and hatred directed at people, so I don't rebuild "the tree of knowledge of good and evil" within.

"I" statements help me start to renew my heart and mind's feelings, sense of injustices, motivations, and sinful or confused attitudes. They help me to move away from judging and hurting others and to become a healer and lover instead.

"I" statements are specifically meant to help me process personal stuff (they move me from judging to truth telling); they don't need to always be spoken to the people I am having difficulty with, but I can speak it to them when prompted by God. There is grace, and so I don't have to confront everyone who offends me to demand justice.

Holiness

Since the NT is written to the "holy ones" and all the letters have much advice, wisdom, and correction regarding sinful acts, this means their actions weren't always holy but they themselves were holy in God's eyes. Therefore, they are in a holy position because of their faith in Jesus, since God dwells within them, but they need to become holy in their actions. For those of us who consider ourselves Jesus' disciples we can't make ourselves holy independently of God, but we can make our actions holy[23] through faith in and cooperation with the Holy Spirit.

---

[23] Cf. 1 Peter 1:13-15

So, when the NT writers call us to be holy they mean to become healthy in our thinking, believing, attitudes, behaviors, deeds, speech, and acts. This is the meaning of the verse, "Be Holy for I (God) am Holy," that Peter mentions in his first letter. True holiness comes from being dependent on and trusting in God through His grace. It isn't something we just decide to do and become through our own energy.

The aim of holiness is to live healthily. That means doing what I was hardwired for. Jesus commanded me to live out the Golden Rule which says, "Do to others what I want done to myself." This does not mean I assume that what makes me happy is the same thing that makes others happy. Everyone gets to decide what makes themselves happy. But the Golden Rule does mean that I love others unconditionally because I want to be loved unconditionally. This means that I love people whether they do good, do bad, or are apathetic.

If I am to obey Jesus' commands, like the Golden Rule, and not just call Him "Lord" without doing what He asks, then I need to be free enough to do so. I need to draw from Jesus' peace and energy without pressure and force. The devil quotes the same scriptures to me too, but they become law—not liberating truth—because the devil has a mean, disrespectful, restless, pressurized, and an "I got a whip in my hand so do what I say" dark energy about him. Jesus though is gentle, kind, respectful, and asks us to obey Him with a peaceful yet authoritative energized presence. The devil appeals to my guilt, fear, pride and desires for perfectionism, whereas Jesus appeals to that part of me that cares and believes in Him and wants His will done.

I can adopt either one of these energies when I attempt to speak (to myself or others), or when I attempt to motivate myself or other peoples' actions. But if I choose to heed or copy the devil's voice I won't ever keep Jesus' commands gently, and I will drown in negativity: with "it's my right" kind of anger; with "it isn't fair," "poor-me," "woe-is-me," and "I can't do it" thinking; with sour and bitter emotions and attitudes; and with no healthy actions to show for any of it. But when I choose Jesus' peaceful clean energy poured into my heart by listening to Jesus' voice (and speaking to myself like He does with me), His peace will come with power so that I will be able to love like He commands. This does not come from intellectual analyzing of things—it comes from caring, faith, wisdom, and the desire to love people like Jesus does.

How do I know who I am listening to or copying? When I ask people to "believe in Jesus as Lord and Savior," do I do so in a hard, abrasive, overly serious tone of, "You better or you are damned," or "You got no choice in the matter"? If so, then I have Jesus confused with someone else. Jesus has healthy speech, warmth, kindness, clean energy and emotions. He respects that people have a choice in the matter of His invitations. And He is not abrasive, hard, mean, or over-bearing.

I need to process my thoughts and emotions in prayer, reasoning together with God, and get to the place where I call Jesus "Lord" with healthy respect, firmness, and peace with who He is. I need to live with a clean conscience, knowing Him as caring, loyal and kind; not giving people the impression that He is heartlessly demanding, spiteful, judgmental, or spiritually constipated.

Fully believing in Jesus means I see Him as He is portrayed in the NT. It means that I have not laminated a darkness on to Him in my mind. It means that I respect Him as Leader, Shepherd, Brother, King, Lord, Anointed One, Son of God, and as fully God and as fully Man. It means to not buy any lies from the devil about Jesus. When we do this, Jesus' promise that living waters would flow within us becomes true.

Submission and Resisting:

What does "submitting to God and resisting the devil" so that "the devil will flee" mean? It is very important in cementing victory in the spiritual life. The "submission" part means the following: we accept and commit to God's will (the good, the bad and the ugly in life); we desire God's will; we pray for God's will; and we say yes to God's will above our own wills—whole-heartedly, firmly, not superficially, and not flimsily. The "resisting the devil" part means we say, "I don't need your empty promises Satan," countering his lies with strategic truth. And we say yes to grace and to Jesus, who gives His Holy Spirit generously. We need to ask the Holy Spirit to overcome our sin for there to be victory. Out of submission comes self-discipline and self-control.

Many people, myself included, have believed they don't have self-discipline or self-control because of years of failure. But after we have dismantled and uprooted "the tree of knowledge of good and evil" within, then giving up the lie (in prayer) that we can't practice self-control or discipline, needs to be done. And then we need to start practicing using them as much as we are able to.

Healthy submission to God, spouses, and human authority means that in the face of persecution, hurts, violence, abuse, anger, and conflict we do not return evil for evil, or hurt for hurt, but follow the way of non-violence as a pathway to conflict resolution. This is what Jesus did.

We can't submit to God in our own strength. God strengthens us when we recognize we can't do it without Him and we ask Him to help us. When we begin to judge God, we lose grace, strength, and fellowship; we come under the devil's influence unable to love supernaturally.

Giving up commitments to use anger, bad attitudes, and energies is one way to resist the devil. And committing to the opposite of the vices, namely virtues (healthy attitudes), by submitting to God in prayer will help bring about healthy behaviors.

Exalting myself or my opinions over that which is written in the NT Scriptures is very unhealthy for me as a child of God. It means I have cut myself off, or am in the process of cutting myself off, from hearing God speak powerfully to me for my comfort, health, direction, and discipline (correction). And so I miss out on peace, grace, friendship, learning, and intimacy with God that comes through faith in Jesus. It also means I am not fully submitting to God, that I will have problems "resisting the devil," and he will not flee from me like I would desire.

5 Expanding My Understanding On How To Dismantle The Unwanted Tree Within Me

I observed one morning that when I prayed rote prayers like the Lord's Prayer, the Serenity Prayer, and especially the Prayer to the Holy Spirit, that I said them with the expectation that all the unpleasant attitudes, the negative emotions, and the dark energy streams inside of me would somehow not be felt anymore. I prayed them because I feared this darkness and what it could do; whenever it peeped out I tried to push it back down. Realizing that praying this way is unhealthy, is half the problem. I realized later that I needed to give up this expectation in my heart too. Attempting to push the darkness down within us is unhealthy, because it keeps "the tree of knowledge of good and evil" intact, hidden, and very powerful.

The truth is—if I don't allow myself to feel the unpleasant attitudes, the negative emotions, the dark energy streams when present (such as selfishness, greed, pride, coveting, envy, wanting to use people, etc.), then I will encounter these obstacles:

1. I won't be able to process them and get rid of them for good,
2. I am saying no to the pleasant attitudes, the positive emotions, and the light energy (grace) too, because they, along with the dark energy, come from the same source—my heart. I realized that if I watch over my emotions like a moral policeman suppressing negative emotions and bad energy all the time, then I would be disorientated, numb, out of touch with reality.
3. I end up being a hypocrite, acting as if everything is okay, but my heart doesn't change and I only look clean on the outside.

If I don't suppress my negative emotions, then they are going to be felt by me—and that is a healthy thing because then God and I can process them together. That does not mean I speak this negativity out or act it out against people, because then I'd hurt them by it. But when I deal with it wisely, as I have learned and discuss in this book, I have found it will eventually be cleaned up one area at a time. Ignoring my negative emotions and trying to just focus on the positive ones is like avoiding cleaning the inside of a cup; the whole cup remains dirty—just like Jesus warned us to keep from doing.[24]

It is not wise to rush processing our emotions. Sometimes we can quickly process them but not always. The less congested we are with things like malice, resentments, and making judgments the quicker we will recognize where we are at and what needs to be done, because Christ's light shines more fully into our consciences and through us.

However, as the renewal process advances, sometimes we will get frustrated because of our

---

[24] Cf. Luke 11:39

confusion. This is a healthy sign that we are moving in the right direction. Just stepping back and shaking off the confusion like water off a duck's back is the healthiest thing to do—or keep walking through the fog until we come to see the truth more clearly. We don't have to control and understand everything. Recommitting to trust in Jesus to save us from our sins, and to walk in grace through faith (not sight) will give us clarity of mind and real renewal—more so than trying to wrestle with it all. Understanding comes gradually.

When I am aware of the "sin nature" (the "flesh" within me that uses anger or self-pity to get it's way), I know it can't submit to the Spirit and it frustrates love. It is sinful, corrupt, selfish, and insecure and tries to push me away from living humbly and with self-control. Knowing the "sin nature" won't die in this life keeps me humble because I know it is within me, as it is within every other fallible human being. I come to see that I am no better than anyone else; we all have this "flesh" to deal with no matter how spiritual we are or how hard we try to live holy lives. This book is my attempt to show how I am learning to have victory over the "sin tree" and the "sin nature" one battle at a time.

We know we have a stronghold of sin when it is compulsive, hard to shake off, and threatens to hurt our relationship(s). The first line of attack is confession, and the second is repentance in prayer. Then when the stronghold is removed, the heart and mind need to be renewed and softened in those areas (as per the strategies found in chapters 3 and 4).

Practicing the Golden Rule is not *fully possible* until the roots and branches of the "tree of knowledge of good and evil" are uprooted or dismantled within us. But when we have any resentments against anybody, then we will have problems practicing the Golden Rule and bad fruit will continue to grow. Pride won't be defeated until we forgive whoever we need to from our hearts.

It should be noted that confession and repenting in prayer deals with our ties to the past (distant and recent). And while they present as struggles in all contexts found in this book, they help us deal with our guilt and baggage for good. Confession and repenting in prayer opens our eyes to a healthier way to process our emotions, beliefs, and thinking. Jesus is that better and healthier way. Jesus helps us aim so high that the negative, self-pitying, demanding, self-centered, perfectionistic, angry and judgmental tree-structure is replaced with love, positivity, kindness, generosity, and gentleness by the Holy Spirit.

Jesus said, "Those who keep His words, are truly His disciples. They will know the truth, and the truth will set them free."[25] This is a promise, and Jesus always keeps his promises provided we hold onto them. When the past is dealt with through confession and repentance in prayer we are forgiven and given new opportunities to grow the fruit of the Spirit. As we forge ahead, we

---

[25] Cf. John 8:31-32

continue to confess and repent in prayer; we renew the attitudes and expectations of our minds with Jesus' presence; his teaching, truth, grace, commands, and promises and we choose to put them into practice daily. The NT Scripture has so much truth, and all of it will help us to be set free through the Spirit's leading. When we get stuck, which can happen depending on how strong the battle is, just asking the Holy Spirit to heal our minds and then resting in His faithfulness and grace is key to victory. God will never leave us nor forsake us. He will complete the work He began in us.

5.2: Diagnosing Self-Pity

Self-pity can be felt in reaction to events that happen in our lives because of our expectations, but it can also be used as a means to grow "the tree of knowledge of good and evil" within us.

When we try to immaturely use self-pity to get our own way then it works together with our demanding nature and pride in growing the rest of "the tree of knowledge of good and evil" in our lives. When we pray about it with Jesus' help (as suggested in chapter 6.3), God will shrink the stronghold of self-pity in our lives to manageable terms.

Having dealt with the stronghold of self-pity, we can still feel remnants of self-pity in certain situations, but it doesn't have the brute force it did when it was a stronghold. To keep this weaker form of self-pity in check we need to embrace grace, truth, and loving the people who somehow trigger our self-pity. When we allow people to draw out of us our worst attitudes we need to regroup with wisdom.

Mourning is natural when real injustices happen, but everyone will have different opinions on what violations or injustices are. A healthy spiritual person won't go to a place of self-pity, anger, or coercion; rather they go the extra mile, care for others, are unselfish, and love people.

Self-pity can spring from believing things are unfair and so it easily blames God. Self-pity can spring from selfishness. Self-pity can spring up in all our relationships at church, at work, and at play: in friendships, in families, and in marriages. Self-pity springs from things that are denied us.

Grace and truth helps to fortify us from giving into a self-pity that could possibly develop into an ugly stronghold.

When we are asked to do things that are altruistic in nature the natural thing to do, if we are unfamiliar with love, is to pout, sulk, and become full of self-pity. This is because our pride is hurt, and we were asked to do something that we know we ought to have done without being asked. This can be very ugly when not hidden from others.

When I feel a powerful sense of self-pity, in the context of hurt feelings (when people seemingly ignore me or are cold towards me), I know I am struggling with conceit too. I am also struggling with trust issues, and I am tempted to judge, manipulate, and unkindly demand things all out of pride. I need to pray about my conceit, along with all of the baggage outlined here, to get free from self-pity. Yes, self-pity can be triggered by conceit (see how to deal with this in chapter 6.9).

As one learns to diagnose where self-pity is coming from the next steps are to find healing with God's help in prayer. Yes, there have been remarkable results for me, but usually they are followed by newer challenges. For me, being so full of pride for the longest time, the results have seemed very gradual. Giving time for the Holy Spirit to help me process my beliefs, feelings, thinking, and attitudes, and allowing myself time to grow in positive virtues is very important. Self-pity often springs up on many fronts in our relational lives and it will take time to sort the triggers out. But because God's promises do route the enemy's strongholds, when we cooperate with God through grace and truth, it gets sorted out eventually.

5.3: Dismantling The Foolish Roots Of The Tree: Healing Broken Relationships

When we aren't in a relationship with God—and many times when we are, but not perfectly—then it means that we can be committed to certain foundational beliefs that are not in line with who God is (Love) and that distort how we see our neighbors and ourselves. These beliefs are often very foolish and judgmental, and often cause us to sin against God and in such a way that some of our relationships tend to go sour. These beliefs help to form the roots of "the tree of knowledge of good and evil" within us. These faulty and foolish beliefs need to be replaced with freeing truths. The sins that spring from these beliefs need to be confessed to God and repented from in faith too. It is not enough to just forgive ourselves; God needs to forgive us too. And with this forgiveness comes healing, as we cooperate with God in renewing our minds and hearts through grace, truth, and relationship with Jesus.

There is always room for growth and resurrection in our relationships. Foolish beliefs, sin, and guilt are the source of our broken relationships with God and others. Most of the healing we can experience comes from dealing healthily with our foolish beliefs, sin, and guilt through repentance, forgiveness, grace and truth. Not wanting to love or pay the price to love brings us guilt, weakens our connection with God, and grows "the tree of knowledge of good and evil" within us. Deciding to commit to love through God's forgiveness and grace, and caring about people instead of resenting them, helps to mend our relationships with God and others. If we refuse to love people, then we refuse to love God.

Another part to being foolish is believing lies that lead to feeling that things are always unfair that cause us to not have victory and love like we are intended to. Believing that things are always unfair really is a BIG root to so much jealousy and judgment and leads to a parasitical nature.

On a different note, I became wounded during a traumatic event as a young child at a track meet I attended at a huge stadium in South Africa. I felt my world falling apart and got stuck in a lot of trauma by embracing the fear of being screamed at for not being on time for an event, and for not living up to the thousands of spectators' expectations. I did not want to feel the pain I felt on that day again, so I foolishly committed to being early for events so no one would scream at me again. I also started to carry the emotional load of meeting the expectations of any crowd that gathered around me. In a conversation with a friend, I realized that no one is going to very likely scream at me. I confronted the fear and a lot of my anxiety left. I also let go of trying to meet large crowds' unspoken expectations. I am now able to be more compassionate to those who come my way daily requiring some of my time.

Believing lies, committing sin, being unforgiving, coveting, being jealous, telling lies, judging, and being committed to our pride, can all be walls that keep God and others out of our lives and creates a senseless life. Putting our faith humbly in Jesus and receiving His grace and truth are the start and foundation from which to live, forgive, be forgiven, and successfully give up sin strongholds. When we forgive the agents of our hurts, or wounds, then we are healed spiritually. Without forgiveness there is no freedom.

Relationships can break down because we believe lies. Adam and Eve's relationships with God, and each other, were damaged because they began believing the lies from the devil. To dismantle the tree structure within I need to let God, through prayer, expose the lies I believe and replace them with truth. The truth always sets free. I also need to repent in prayer from acting out the sin that comes from the lies I believed.

I have come to realize that I can't rush this process. And it's a good idea to pray through my baggage in whatever areas God brings to my mind to establish a firm foundation from which I see God as good, kind, patient, and compassionate. In doing this I slowly grow in the peace Jesus promises. When I've prayed to God—renouncing my idols that I previously had put in place of God—then I need to remember that I did so because I wanted peace, and the idols I chose could not satisfy my hunger and thirst for this goodness. Often, I wrongly look for peace with certain parts of my body. If I have compulsive-indulging in my life, for instance, then feeding the location that most gives pleasure when eating is where I am seeking my peace. If this is the case, then giving up seeking peace in that place through prayer is the place to start; I then must invite God's peace into my life instead.

It is fitting that when we worship God one of the things we can call Him is our "Prince of Peace" and accept Him in faith. But all this can be done in vain if we don't nurture our relationships with God. To do this we need to seek God with all our hearts, and this means spending time with God: speaking with Him, listening to Him, and giving up other distractions and pursuits that would seek to supplant our relationship with God. Journaling is the best way to nurture our relationship with God (as discussed earlier in the book). Reading theology or self-help books do not count as friendship time spent with God, even though they can be beneficial in many ways. Relationship is not only knowing about somebody, but interacting with somebody in a meaningful and connecting way.

Jesus said that He is the True Vine and that we are the branches. His life and grace should flow into us. When we abide in Him then His life flows into that God shaped vacuum that has an appetite and thirst for God. We must abide in Him, and with Him in us, if we are to bear good fruit. To abide in Jesus means to humble oneself and jettison, through prayer, the idols we are aware of so the life and grace of Jesus can fully sustain us. Next, to abide in Jesus means our allegiance belongs to Him and not to the world, the devil, or the "flesh." When God teaches us something we need to hold onto it. When people tell us something contrary to the Good News then that is the world's message that we ought to reject lovingly, gently, patiently, respectfully, and caringly; not judgmentally, coldly, meanly, angrily, hatefully, in ugliness, with hostility or cold hard walls going up.

When "the tree of knowledge of good and evil," matures it leads to much idol worship and has competed for my devotion and time that I would otherwise have given to God. In dismantling this horrible structure through faith in Jesus, and with the tools developed in this book, I am growing in my relationship with God and people.

Throughout each day, I can encounter situations that baffle me, and seem to dry up the soft places in my heart. I turn into a cold, dry, judgmental and abrasive person interiorly even though outwardly I wear masks to keep the peace or to do damage control. When this happens I find that talking to God about it in conversation is where to start. It is always the place to start. God may point out many different things to me: to deal with an unforgiving nature in my heart; to face the fears triggered by certain lies I believed that need to be replaced with truth; to healthily own my anger because of injustices (which is not sinful); or to invite grace more fully into my life. If these don't fully help, then a healthy thing to do is to go deeper in prayer with Jesus' light in our hearts, and use the tools He has provided and as He directs. The tools I mention here are all found in the NT Scriptures, but brought together to provide a focused strategy to conquer sin and to grow in loving others.

For a long time my main approach to prayer had been to ask for stuff only when I got into trouble; the rest of the time was just having long conversations with myself—relying on what I knew and believed, mixed up with fear, blind spots, and often being "out to lunch" or off topic when it came to what needed to be dealt with. When this happened, I found the thing to do was to give up trying to heal myself by my own energy and instead trust God's promises and invitation to hear His voice.

I now realize that instead of having a conversation with myself all day long I can have one with the Holy Spirit. And you know what? The ideas and truths that come to mind when I do so are so freeing, calming, and needed that I know they have come from God; no amount of analyzing, scratching my head, and taking leaps in logic have ever given me something so wholesome to hang onto like what the Holy Spirit gives. I have a choice: either a stagnant pond or a life-giving stream flowing into my interior life.

We all need a focus to have direction in life. Knowing, listening to, and being able to sense the tone, the energy, the attitude, the grace, the truth, and the authority of Jesus' voice brings us a peace the world cannot give. It gives us the correct and healthy disposition necessary to walk in "the valley of the shadow of death." When we start talking to ourselves like Jesus does to us, then we really start loving ourselves healthily.

In becoming aware of the connections between the building blocks of "the tree of knowledge of good and evil" I find it best to look at my bad fruit and ask what fears motivate them. I ask the Holy Spirit what lies motivate or keep the tree structure together through fear within me. Once the connections are realized it is time to dismantle them through grace, strategic prayer, and truth. This involves confessing my sins, bad attitudes, bad energy and fears, and repenting in prayer with grace from them, by working upwards through the Tree Diagram. This keeps the guessing, frustration, and time frame to a minimum, and helps me to find and dismantle the real motivations and roots of my sin strongholds, to find freedom to love others more deeply.

When confusion and carnal energy manifest themselves repeatedly in the present, then know that either the past is not fully dealt with or there is something in the present not right. When we have problems navigating a relationship then it can perhaps be that we are embracing unhealthy beliefs about the person in question. If our beliefs lead us to unwholesome energy directed towards the person, then we need to examine our beliefs with Jesus' help. If we are compulsively judging, then focusing on a truth (i.e. the line between good and evil goes through each person's soul and does not divide communities, groups, political parties, or religions) may do away with the inner conflict.

In order to remain sane, one needs to focus on healthy goals. When one's focus is on old lies or negative tapes then one will stumble and fall and not execute strongly and masterfully what needs to be done. These tapes or lies can form when we are most impressionable. Like when we are feeling rejected, hurt, ridiculed and hated and the devil or a willing instrument of his malice comes to rob us of our hope, kind energy and destiny.

When we have been hurt or wounded that is when the devil promises stuff that seems justified; however, the devil's promises are always empty, and rob us of our true humanity. Intense fear and confusion go together and cloud our judgment; we are lead to think we are saving ourselves by holding onto the power and promises from the dark side. The devil promises power and tries to justify our sense of injustice or unfairness to win us over to permanent resentments. This needs to be prayed through thoroughly for grace, truth, healing and freedom to flourish and thrive instead.

5.4: Visiting Sins On Children By Parents

It must be said that in this place of foolishness that causes broken relationships with God and people, that our parents, family members, and teachers have a very great influence for good and bad in our lives. For instance, when a parent foolishly tries to correct or judges a child the way they themselves were wrongly directed by their own parents.

Their child can become confused, projecting the evil judgments that are visited on them by their parents onto the way they see God judging people. And, because they see God in this unhealthy fashion, they land up judging people, situations, and acts in unhealthy ways in part as acts of false worship. This can be a root that causes unhealthy compulsive-judging and prejudices in the child on into adulthood when not corrected with wisdom, kindness, patience, and caring.

Praying through such strongholds in healthy ways like those suggested in this book is key to dismantling them. I do not suggest that we bash and blame our parents, but we shouldn't minimize their sins either. There is room for kindness, care, and forgiveness in all of our relationships when we seek it out. Having said this, fear and confusion will arise when we challenge such strongholds. Holding onto Jesus' kindness and promises are key to navigating out of such interior and relational darkness.

6 Diagnosing & Healing Fear

When a relationship with God is broken in some way, fear comes into play; we too often listen to the devil's lies and don't recognize God's truth because of disconnects in our thinking. Fear is a building block to "the tree of knowledge of good and evil" within us. Fear has so much destructive power and can move me to where a sane person would not tread.

Satan uses fear to try to paralyze me with this lie: "God is not good enough to get you through your challenges." This lie robs me from going the extra mile and, if I'm not careful, from living out this truth: "I can do all things through Christ Jesus who strengthens me."[26] Recognizing the lie when I have it and giving it up in prayer through faith, whether it is a conscious or subconscious belief, and embracing the corresponding truth is the healthy path to take.

In the diagram below two continuums are illustrated, and in between these is where spiritually healthy individuals can embrace grace, love and forming real community. As we become more fear driven out of insecurity we will move away from the center to the right towards legalism. As we become more fear driven by shame we will move away from the center to the left towards rebellion. Unreasonable fears are always rooted in lies about our relationships, self-images, and identities.

But when we practice grace and humility—which means "truth and not judging" is embraced—we are moved away from the extremes of legalism and rebellion towards the center. And when we experience grace in the form of caring we can easily move to the center where real community exists.

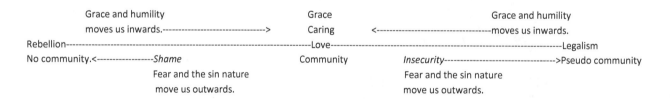

The "sin nature" within each of us provides the energy and pull to move us away from the center towards the extremes along either continuum—through fear, shame, insecurity, and anger—when we let it. These extremes of rebellion and legalism aren't real solutions, but are perversions of safe and healthy communities.

All Christian communities on earth are not perfect. When problems and injustices happen within them and we don't rely on God's truth, grace and love, we move towards either rebellion or

---

[26] Philippians 4:13

legalism, because then we don't fully grant forgiveness, grace, mercy, love and tolerance to others within those communities. Or perhaps the community we may have belonged to did not grant us enough grace and mercy either. No community can really seem safe to those who are hurt or have been threatened with shame, because trust only comes when people know they are cared for.

Rebellion means we don't want rules (or the rules from our former community), and out of anger we want self-determination. And so we become the captains of our own ships, and maybe even toy with the idea of being our own gods. We may do so because we want to be strong in the eyes of others, not show our fears, or not be the objects of shame and ridicule. Some who slowly rebel against real community begin to play around with the idea of hating their former home and what it stands for.

When we practice legalism, it means we feel insecure. This moves us to seeking security through rule-keeping which leads us to measuring performance and focusing on outward appearances. Rules slowly become more important than the people in the community.

The rules will initially look something like fairness or love, but as time goes by the practices, energy and interpretations will focus more on conformity based in fear, than the unconditional love found in genuine, healthy communities. The rule keeping will be done more and more in a spirit of apathy or in some, engender anger, pressure and fear.

Infraction of the rules cause guilt in the offenders, but may draw anger, judging, meanness, and hatred from the legalistic members of the community. And the possibility of discipline or rejection from this colder group of leaders prompts a "try harder" and "do more" mentality from the "guilty" offenders, to avoid pain and judging. Pseudo community develops as a result of those willing to do anything to belong; their insecurity making them see obeying rules as the way to belong.

But no person is perfect, so those people in the legalistic group will do a lot of pretending; resulting in plenty of hypocrisy within, and the pseudo community will persist in its unhealthy relating style.

Legalism holds people to anal standards that would be difficult for most of us to maintain. People caught in the vise of legalism are often full of self-pity, anger, and fear—miserable when something challenges their way of doing things.

Only grace and humility, in the context of truth, can free us from the deadly mixture of legalism and rebellion. Freedom and the herd instinct are very strong God-given drives within our makeup. When trauma or threats come our way, then our reactions can become knit together in the form of rebellion and legalism; we are willing to do anything in our power to avoid the hurt, to rid ourselves of confusion, or to stop threats to our identity, self-esteem, and security.

This all needs to be addressed with God's wisdom and grace.

I had both rebellion and legalism in my makeup because of how two authority figures (both teachers in grade school) tried to humiliate me by making me an example. I realized that I needed to forgive them and learn what healthy and unhealthy herd instincts are.

Healthy herd instinct happens when the other members of the herd are prepared to listen to one member's wisdom, provided they hold to truth and grace. Each member of the herd has something to contribute, but is also dependent on the input from the rest of the herd and welcomes input when needed.

To have freedom means one is not being compulsive in one's behavior, being coerced, being threatened, or being forced by others to be loyal through fear, demonizing, or ostracizing. In healthy groups one stays connected because of mutual respect, honor, and care; and because one is loved, valued, and seen as having dignity.

Note: The above discussion deals with fear that is present in conforming to the maxims of the herd. But when there is no fear felt, or a person isn't in touch with her or his fear, then a person may be in denial pretending nothing has happened. They are stuck, and need help getting unstuck.

6.2: Different Fears

We are all hungry and thirsty people, with earthly and spiritual appetites. When we don't know how our needs or wants are going to be met, then we can have plenty of fears.

Fear pushes us either to God, or it pushes us to solving our own problems through our own know-how, creativity and energy, independently of Him. When we choose unbelief and ignore God we use pride to meet our physical, emotional, and spiritual needs. Simply giving up the fear and believing God for His ever-helping presence and provisions in prayer is the wise path to take; it helps uproot "the tree of knowledge of good and evil" within us. The less fear within us the more we are rooted in love. It is what we do with our fears that matters.

There are many different fears: of having to pay the price for certain actions; of having to wait for people; of being inconvenienced; of not getting attention or recognition; of not getting our way; of having to work, sacrifice, or sweat to earn a living; or of having to commit to loving a person or group of people we don't like.

Fears of the unknown can also be powerful motivators, especially in creating a judgmental attitude within us. If we are unhealthily angry, it is often because fear produces vices, that in turn produces more anger and all sorts of judgments in our head. If we have a severed relationship with God, we attempt to do many things apart from Him out of fear: we seek to give ourselves the credit for the happy results in our life; we blame God when stuff goes wrong; and we use methodologies that are not only unhealthy, but are harmful and independent from God's grace. Such actions negate the supernatural, unconditional love—also known as "grace"—from our lives.

God *really* wants to help us so He does everything in His power to restore us to Himself. The fears we have need to be dealt with: through God's presence, grace, truth, and promises; through prayer; and through walking with Jesus in faith.

Giving up our fears in prayer is done by meeting them head-on: confronting them with common sense truth, biblical truth, God's promises; and intellectually and emotionally embracing God's unconditional love or grace. Making a list of fears and praying through them is key. Love casts out all unreasonable fears, with truth that is positive, humble, respectful of boundaries, healthy in belief and thinking, and based on the loving touch of God.

This does not mean that we ought to act naively or like parasites towards the people in our lives in order to receive or feel love; rather love sets us free.

It is not wise to pray, "Jesus, I wish you were my meaning and peace (or life and joy)" in this context. But it is wise to regularly make lists of unreasonable fears and pray them out loud (as shown in chapters 3 and 4), and then to invoke the promises found in Scripture that push our fears away. When we do the latter, we are opening the doors of grace and faith, putting to death our fears by changing what we believe, and giving God His rightful place at the center of our lives.

It is true that love casts out all fear. When we know that we are loved, then the accusations in our heads that question that love are easily deflected with our shields of faith or trust. Fear is crippling when it turns into self-pity, worry, cowardice and conceitedness. Knowing who God is, and who we are in Him, is very important when it comes to listening to our intuitions. Listening to our spirits, when they say trust or don't trust a person in our lives, will give us peace and remove fears that otherwise could drive us crazy or make us paranoid. Listening to the Holy Spirit is also important along with reading and understanding the Holy Scriptures. All relationships are based on trust, or the lack thereof.

Giving up a fear, by committing to God's grace, and saying to the fear, "I give you up through God's grace," is wiser than just trying to say to it "no." The former is freeing, whereas the latter tries to use force. Saying "no" to fear usually ends in a power struggle with the flesh, by giving it a stronger "in-our-face" presence and allowing more temptation in our backyards (spiritually speaking). Making this switch in how we speak to our fears and sins can be life altering.

6.3: Healing Fear And Self-Pity

Fear of things not being fair can lead to compulsively demanding them to be so. Fear is not a good motivator and can lead to using immoral means to further our goals. Fear needs to be confessed, repented from in prayer, and replaced with seeking to live with healthy energy instead.

For instance, fear can motivate the use of self-pity because of loss, supposed unfairness, and possible broken promises. We can go around searching for healthy ways to feed our appetites, but when they aren't satisfied by God, spouses, parents, children, friends, coworkers, employers or people who cross our paths every day for whatever reasons, then either we move to sorrow or self-pity because of the seeming unfairness. If we move to sorrow (that we put this expectation upon another person and feel sad for the perceived loss of their caring for us), then we will move to peace, love and self-control and won't look for unhealthy ways to get our hunger and thirsts met. If we move to self-pity, then we will try to control others or whatever is at our disposal to get our own way. These thoughts are summarized in the diagram (by reading down from the top):

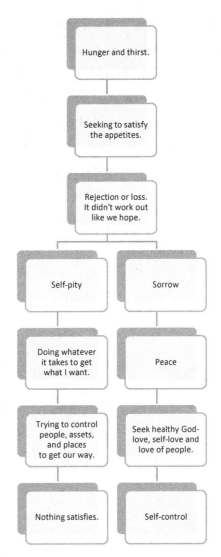

Self-pity believes we are all alone and no one cares for us and our cause—not even God. Self-pity cuts away at our faith in people and God. Self-pity leads to despair, anger, and abandoning relationships that do not satisfy.

Jesus said that He had "food" that His disciples knew nothing about. His "food" was to do the will of His Father. Jesus is saying that there are real rewards like meaning, purpose, happiness, and fulfillment in healthily seeking to do and accomplish what God desires from us; and these are more satisfying than instant gratification or earthly hunger and thirsts. Love does not seek its own in any relationship. We are wired for altruism, nobility, and honor because we are made in the image of God—despite being infected with a sinful nature. The "sin nature" opposes the noble side God grants each of us at conception.

There is a real difference in godly sorrow versus self-pity. Sorrow is selfless, rational sadness. Self-pity is self-centered, irrational sadness. Self-pity can lead to suicide, whereas sorrow leads to giving our lives so that others can live. Self-pity goes the way of possibly taking life; whereas sorrow feels sad for others and seeks to give life instead of erecting walls.

People who can't take a perfectly good "no" for an answer to a request will sulk and have plenty of self-pity if they don't take by force what they covet or demand. Learning to accept awkward people, situations, and unfairness in life, and giving people the right to refuse will transform our selfish attitude into humility and love. I know that when we have massive bouts of self-pity in situations, then the healthy thing to do is trade in that self-pity for love. And this is done by dismantling all the Sin-Conduit Structures that contain selfishness in "the tree of knowledge of good and evil" within me. In doing this my self-pity shrinks to a manageable size. For the longest time I was in love with myself and I realized that this needed to change. I needed to embrace Jesus' command to, "Love the Lord my God with all my heart, soul, and strength; and to love my neighbor as myself."[27] For the longest time I was my own idol, and I worshipped myself religiously. Thankfully, Jesus changed this with my cooperation through prayer starting with the Sin-Conduit Structure illustrated below:

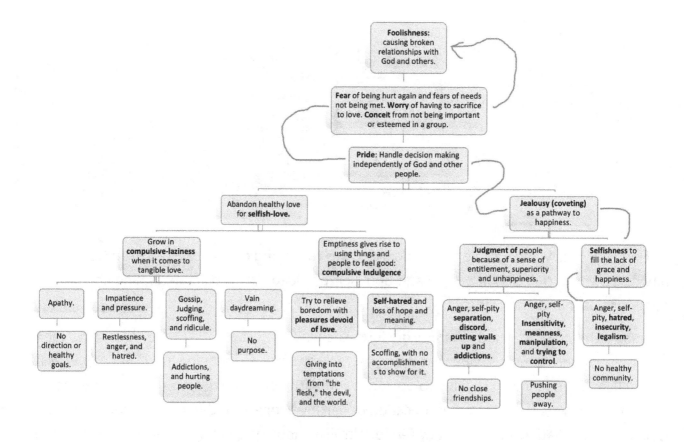

---

[27] Cf. Mark 12:30-31

This Sin-Conduit Structure has the following Sin-Anatomy Table:

Self-pity	Selfishness	Coveting & Jealousy	Pride	Fear & Conceit	Foolishness
	<=	<=	<=	<=	<= Cause and Effect
Debilitating self-pity. Having the gall to use self-pity to manipulate, pressure, and demand stuff from people.	Been selfish most of my life to the core. When others get opportunities I've tried to out maneuver them to get the coveted prizes.	I've not been very charitable or happy for people who have what I want. Tried to wrestle God into giving me more power, more goodies, more opportunities.	I'm committed to being first in so many contexts in my life.	Always afraid of being left out, or missing an opportunity. Afraid I might have to give of myself.	Cared plenty for humanity, but very little for individual people. Saw loving people as too burdensome. Am in love with myself.
I treated so many people this way…					
Confession & Repenting in Faith =>	=>	=>	=>	=>	

Prayer to dismantle this Sin-Conduit Structure:

Lord God I confess that I have a stronghold of self-pity in my life. I know that the way to tackle it is to understand what is beneath it. And you have convinced me that part of the structure contains my selfishness. Lord God I confess that I have been self-centered and selfish most my life. Not a caring person, but selfish to the core and full of jealousy when the opportunities present themselves. Please forgive me Lord Jesus. I am in the wrong and regret it deeply. I admit that this comes from my pride that is committed to being first in all contexts of my life. I remember thinking like this as a small child in South Africa, while in university in Canada, and the way I have lived life up until now, when I was not practicing your presence Lord Jesus. I admit that I have conceit and fear too. And I did everything to put myself first; including not caring for other people most of my life because I saw loving other people as too difficult—which was a lie. Lord God this stems from my foolish decision and commitment to being in love with myself. I confess these sins and give them up, with your help and by faith in you Jesus. Thank you. Please help me to renew my mind in this context too, Lord God. I recommit to loving you with all my heart, soul, and strength and to love my neighbor as myself. Thank you for your forgiveness and healing in this area in my life. Amen.

Recognizing a Sin-Conduit Structure in my consciousness, when it rears its ugly head, means I have an opportunity to dismantle it with God's help. I need to repent in prayer from such structures within me and say yes to healthier ways of relating through believing truth over lies. A healthy relationship with God is the only way to conquer and dismantle those deadly or harmful structures within me. It is in the context of relationship with Jesus, community, and prayer where we find positive change.

6.4: Boxed-In By Self-Pity

As children we may have sometimes taken disappointment really hard and cried a lot, with an insensitive parent or teacher making fun of us by calling us hurtful names—perhaps trying to turn us into fully-grown men or women through insults. Our reaction may have been to resist the name calling by saying no to it, but in doing so it created a box that we try to fight our way out of for the rest of our lives or until the truth sets us free.

When a child has the habit of always crying, then the child turned adult may struggle with self-pity, with the expectation that the worst will always happen. This makes a person very negative and needy. The only way out of this box is to give up saying no to the self-pity, and instead give up the crying, and the self-pity itself, in faith and with Jesus' help. We must also forgive the parent or teacher from our hearts. A way to do this is to say, "I accept that you—self-pity—are a part of my old life, but I don't need you right now." And to then pray that you give it up, with Jesus' help through faith. Tell Jesus that His grace is more desirable and that you choose to do His will instead.

We will then have to renew our mind and heart (as discussed in chapter 4). We need to believe that we can maturely handle whatever negative things life throws our way and recognize that, "I can do all things through Christ Jesus who strengthens me."[28] It is our faith that enables us to overcome the world. This quote from St. Paul was intended to give courage to believers who find themselves in difficult situations, but was never meant to be interpreted to mean that we can all run the 100-meter dash in world record time or that we can all make it rich. As we renew our minds on a proper foundation, we will see things that used to throw us for a loop with new eyes. We will handle fears, threats, and broken relationships with wisdom and gentleness.

6.5: Self-Pity And Complaining

The diagram below has its genesis in the OT story when the Jews complained to, whined against, and criticized Moses and God, and includes what the Holy Spirit has been teaching me about these behaviors in myself. First of all, I now know I can determine what I focus on and think about—both positive and negative. I don't have to be at the mercy of any fallen angel's

---

[28] Philippians 4:13

confusing lies, or anyone else's for that matter, unless I have a compulsive attitude that draws negativity to me.

All the negativity (fear, self-pity, anxiety, and powerlessness) we might feel are inspired by the dark thoughts we think and believe. They are often inserted into our minds by fallen angels and are often hurtful and scary. We can either tune into them or turn away from them. All the positive, warm, and respectful thoughts inserted into our minds are done in cooperation with the Holy Spirit. We can either tune into them or turn away from them. All our feelings are from what we focus on. If we rid ourselves from certain negative thoughts, then the feelings we have from them will also go away (provided we didn't start to believe one or more of the lies behind them). Below is a fork in the road diagram that illustrates this (read from the top down).

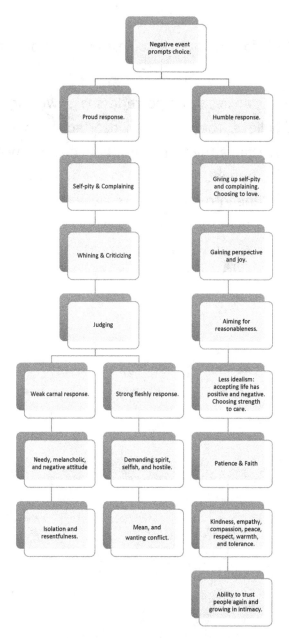

I get to choose where I want to go in my mind; no one else can decide this for me unless I give them that power. I don't have to own the malicious codes the devil puts into my mind unless I choose to agree with them and live them out. The gateway to darkness is through self-pity and complaining, and the more often we go there the more it will accelerate into a judgmental attitude. This leads to selfishness until it becomes a negative stronghold of bitterness in our minds and hearts. The gateway to positivity is saying, "I don't need to indulge in self-pity or complaining." When grace is involved, recognizing that things are unfair leads to compassion, as we choose to love others the way we would want to be loved. The more we give up self-pity and complaining the easier it will be to be positive; to love, to be warm, and to be kind until it becomes the default attitude in our hearts and minds. The struggle to think positively will get easier, but we will always have to choose between indulging in self-pity and complaining or giving up self-pity and complaining. The choice is ours.

Over time the connections on the left side of the diagram above can develop into strongholds until they all become blurred together, and we automatically fall into judgmental attitudes when something negative happens. We might find ourselves vacillating between a resentful attitude retreating into isolation, and a demanding, hostile attitude seeking conflict—expecting our "rights" to be met. The former has the attitude of "poor me" and the latter is about being greedy and "getting even." In either case, they have the following qualities:

- They measure out love less than or equal to what other people measure out to them.
- They are insecure and choose to not love those who don't love them.
- They are motivated by fear of rejection and have low self-esteem.
- They don't know their worth in God's eyes.
- They have believed lies that make them more like parasites than lovers.
- They are motivated by a selfish kind of love—lust.
- They hunger for power to control people, the present, and the future. Therefore, they seek knowledge in these areas either from the occult or in prayer to God.
- They have a goal to save face.
- They often view God's love as conditional, God as hard to please, and God as someone who loves you only if you belong to Him or if you have your theological ducks in a row.
- They may believe God only starts to love you once you give Him reign over your life.
- They also believe they ought to only love others once they have fulfilled all the initiation requirements, belong to their sect, cause or particular denomination, and have a "decent track record".
- They often feel they aren't respected when others don't always do as they please (they take things personally).
- They act from the "flesh" and people sense this as inauthentic so their efforts to get respect always fall short.
- They continually blame others and have difficulty seeing the bright side of things and being thankful.

We have to process the stuff that bothers us instead of complaining. And not complaining means not complaining to God either. So what do we do then? It comes down to first confessing and repenting in prayer from our sin, and then using "I" statements to express to God our feelings, hurts, anger, and frustrations instead. We do this in a renewed way without attacking, judging, criticizing, sulking, and complaining. In this way we aren't used by Satan to accuse people before God of doing vile and mean things. And in speaking to and listening to the Holy Spirit He lightens our loads by putting ideas, truths, and wisdom into our thoughts as we reason with Him in friendship; He helps us to process our negativity in healthy ways.

The listening part might seem like foolishness, but it will come naturally to followers of Jesus who are willing to learn and grow in their relationship with God. Books by Brad Jersak and Mark Virkler are good places to start to read about and grow in two-way prayer.

Humble and non-judgmental people have the following qualities:

- They are strong and love lavishly even those who treat them badly.
- They are secure in who they are.
- They have hope.
- They believe the best about everyone else.
- They do not see themselves as being at the capricious mercy of others.
- They do not struggle for power.
- They are not motivated by fear or fear of rejection.
- They do not attempt to use God as a good luck charm—like a crystal ball that predicts the future conveniently for them so they can safely navigate tricky economic uncertainty.
- They trust God with the future and live as much as possible in the present.
- They view God's love as unconditional (i.e. loving them whether or not they do good, do bad, or are apathetic).
- They believe God is merciful: to the righteous and the wicked; to the knowledgeable and the ignorant; and to the wise and the foolish.
- They continually love, and you can be yourself with them.

Giving up self-pity and complaining, and choosing to love instead, leads to perspective, realism, idealism, patience and faith. We will no longer be looking for things to criticize and find wrong with people and this also leads to trusting others more. So what do we look at to live a non-judgmental life? We look at living out the Golden Rule in the context of "grace."

Choosing to gain perspective, and choosing joy (instead of whining) gives us an intuition for relating to others—a connectedness, a trust, a fellowship, with others—that allows us to navigate the ups and downs in life and gives us the ability to forge deeper commitments to each other.

When we judge harshly or are intolerant of another person's conduct as deeply sinful and unacceptable (correctly or incorrectly)—that we happen to do ourselves (knowingly or unknowingly)—then this is commonly known as hypocrisy. But the Bible says that if we have broken one command, then we have broken the whole law. So hypocrisy is more than committing the exact same sin we have judged in another person to be worse than ours; it is committing any sin, and still to have judged. (Note: Judging any person is always wrong, but telling the truth is different than judging). Our behaviors will not be healed until we deal with our hypocrisy by repenting in prayer from it successfully. And that means we need to stop judging others. It is so easy to compartmentalize our perceptions, and when we do so, then we become blind and will hurt a lot of people when given the opportunity to do so. We compartmentalize our thoughts and attitudes and stuff them into boxes and fail to see the connections to other relevant perceptions.

6.6: Healing Fear, Worry, And Pressure

I have wobbled back and forth from being too easy on myself to being too hard on myself most of my adult life. The pressure I put on myself caused a lot of stress; there were health-related repercussions in my body because of what went on in the mind. I learned I couldn't get rid of being hard, angry, and mean with myself by being hard, angry, and mean with myself.

Being hard on others usually means we are hard on ourselves—but not always. There is a "you reap what you sow" kind of justice; if we seek to start loving others like we want to be loved, then we start to grow spiritually and draw positive energy and grace from God. But we need to deal with the old "sin-conduit" tree structures and branches of pressure, meanness, and pride within us through prayer.

Just because one has high standards does not make one hard on oneself. Being mean and exerting angry pressure on oneself means one is hard on oneself. When one is aiming for high standards but is gentle with oneself, then that is not being hard on oneself. Confessing and repenting from being hard on oneself is the way to heal this. When people say we are hard on ourselves then we should examine ourselves with this in mind.

Being hard on oneself is a result of pride, which in turn is a result of fear and worry. When we have fears then we will worry: worry leads to the need to control; control leads to pressure; pressure leads to meanness, anger, and hatred. When we are hard on or mean to ourselves, we will be hard on and mean to others. If we are hard on ourselves, then we will do so in God's throne room too.

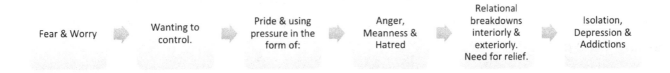

We can be hard on ourselves in one context and not so with others and also we can be easy on ourselves in another context but hard on others. I have found this important to realize so they can be dealt with separately.

I have discerned that I ought not try to manufacture gentleness and heartfelt feelings when I attempt to honestly confess to God and do business with Him in prayer. I need to be real and not magnify or minimize my sins; I need to be truthful and be myself. Being hard on myself was a disposition that needed to be discarded through prayer as I encountered it. And I needed to deal with putting pressure on myself, worrying, and giving into my fears about the future through trust in God's promises. Yes, confession and repentance in prayer are very important, but I needed to deal with my thinking through wisdom and seeing things in new ways.[29] Amen.

If Jesus is gentle with me, then I ought to be gentle with myself and act out of the goodness in my heart. This happens when I renew my mind and heart (as discussed in chapters 3 and 4). I continually need to invite the Spirit of Jesus into my darkness and emptiness: asking Him for healing, asking him to speak into my life; asking questions that can lead to wisdom; and listening to Him in patience. I must know how to pray properly so I can process and deal with issues in my life in a healthy way.

When we put crippling pressure on ourselves or harbor a meanness inside us, then we must realize that it did not get that way overnight. Looking back and admitting to ourselves and God as much as we can remember (along with the pride and worry) is important, because we can then see how the habits formed in us over the years. We can see just how much we need to change our unhealthy beliefs, thoughts, commitments, and idol worship. God will forgive and cleanse us as we trust Him with it. It is very possible to believe the lie that people are mostly pregnant with evil except for ourselves! And therefore believe they deserve what is coming to them. This is judgmental, jaded, proud, and bears the fruit of meanness. God wants to replace such subconscious beliefs with ones that say, "Yes, we deserve the consequences of our sins, but grace checkmates judgments in beautiful ways."

We can be so bound in wanting to control people, being impatient with them, and only caring about ourselves. I'm powerless to control God and others: family, spouse, friends, coworkers, bosses, people on the street, buses, and line-ups. Accepting this powerlessness is key to working on dispensing grace. Controlling others is an illusion.

When we have experienced powerlessness in the past unjustly, then it can trigger frustration, powerlessness, anger, and trying to control people in the present. I once had this problem, but when I forgave those who violated my personal space, then the struggles for control vanished leaving me in peace.

There is no rest or peace in seeking our own wills. Praying for God's will to be done is important to breaking this control mentality. There is peace in seeking God's will, and it moves us away from unhealthy expectations and selfishness. Wanting to control people to save our own lives also comes from the energy found in our "sin nature" and "the tree of knowledge of good and evil" within us.

I determined that my unhealthy thinking comes from accepting the untruths or lies spoken to

---

[29] Cf. My books called *Exploring Faith, Hope & Love*, and *Contrasting Humility and Pride* for new and healthy ways of seeing things

me. I took responsibility for this in repentance and realized that God is willing to help me change by guiding me to new thinking through His truth and grace.

Just praying, "Oh God, I want to change so much. Poor me—I hurt so much. I want to change so much. Amen," will not work, because going no deeper than this leaves everything to God. We must search out what is in our hearts, with God's Light, help, and grace. We must repent in strategic prayer and put to death the weak, "poor me, and I can't do it" attitudes, of worry and fear in our hearts, by resting our faith in God's promises, grace, and truths. There are two actual addiction cycles: one involves putting pressure on oneself, and the other has to do with fear. I talk about them in my book called *Going Deeper With The Twelve Steps*.

6.7: Healing Cowardice

It is true that some people are not afraid to die. I'm not afraid to die—but I was afraid to live. Deep down inside of me I just wanted an easy, cushy, and wimpy passage to Heaven. I did not want to live. I saw life as exhausting and draining. I feared and hated the burdens of life. Basically, I was afraid to live. This is cowardice. It makes us demanding, judgmental, and unloving, because we don't want to pay the price of living life or loving people. This attitude is negative and attracts negativity to us and gives room for demons to work in our lives. When we are not wanting to pay the price, then we take shortcuts. Hence, we have compulsive-laziness, instant gratification, and compulsive-indulging too—just to feel good by numbing out the negative. Not wanting to pay the price for the things that make up our lives leads to not wanting to pay the price to love others.

Crippling fear is the nemesis of courage. Fear is a feeling that can become an attitude causing us to back away weakly from confrontation. If we have negative, poisoned, and hurtful speech, then confrontation is a definite no until we deal with our fear and cowardice. We must renew our minds with a healthy, kind thinking, respectful speech, and relating to others that lends itself to non-violence as a pathway to peace.

Cowardice is produced by lies and fears of being hurt again. Confessing our cowardice as wrong and unhealthy, giving up our fears, and dealing with the hurt so we can act from a place of courage is what Jesus asks us to do. I found it a good idea to pray about my failed past romances in this context, as well as the hurts that happened in all my romances.

6.8: Healing Fear-Induced Meanness

Fear that we can't love people because they do things that trigger hateful meanness in us also should be taken into consideration. To heal this we admit to God and ourselves that we have such fear. We then give up the fear and hateful meanness through faith and with Jesus' help in prayer.

6.9: Healing Conceit

I never knew that I was conceited until I heard what the word *actually* meant. Conceit comes from a fear of not belonging; not being respected or honored, and uses all means to preserve itself. Being conceited means one is self-focused, selfish, or greedy for attention. Seeking esteem has to do with ego. Conceit is rooted in the lie that we don't have self-worth, and that we aren't who God says we are— his child and unconditionally loved by Him.

God used the definition of conceit to illumine a construct within me (illustrated below). I could start to repent from my conceit, and I could find the freedom and love to care and feel empathy for others and connect with them in more meaningful ways.

Conceit out of fear.
- Conceit is a hunger for respect and honor above all else; it creates occasions of rejection from those who don't seem to give them this. It makes us willing to do anything to gain the honor and respect we feel we deserve.
- We either attempt to flatter others to gain honor, or we set up legalistic rules or make demands that are rigid and unreasonable to protect honor. We have plenty of anger and judgment as a result.

Pride & Envy
- Pride is expressed as superiority. This results in pushing people away out of fear. We can't connect with or focus on other people because we are too preoccupied with ourselves or our own agenda. Our superiority leads to hatred, hostility, and anger for others when we are not welcomed; we make manipulative attempts to receive honor.
- Envy is expressed as inferiority. This results in jealousy and a victim mentality. This in turn leads to judging and inflexiblity. Inferiority leads to hatred because we feel boxed-in and confused as to why our rigid boundaries are violated so easily. This is a very negative and limiting attitude and approach to life.

Isolation
- Isolation results in negative, needy attitudes, shallow friendships, little if any intimacy, poor navigation of personal boundaries and violations of other peoples' boundaries. Because of this negativity, one will feel the need to put preasure on oneself to belong, which actually is a form of self-hatred. But this leads to self-pity and shallow, surface-types of relationships.

Being conceited is a fear-based attitude, that works together with both pride and envy, leading to isolation and emptiness.

We break the strongholds of conceit (and address selfishness, pride, and fear) in prayer by confessing it and repenting in prayer when it becomes an issue. Giving up our pride in trying to establish our own honor, respect and justice, and replacing it with seeking true honor and true justice is important. When we choose healthy justice, we have healthy honor; but if we seek honor above justice our moral compass becomes skewed, and we become stuck in self-pity. If we are violent, then we engage in brutality.

We can be conceited in many different relationships and situations in our lives, so when our conceit tries to assert itself repeatedly, we confess it to God, repent in prayer as needed, and each time renew our minds with Jesus' truths, commands, promises, teachings, and unconditional love and grace. We begin to see the world and people differently through the eyes of grace.

To renew the mind, we must remember that our self-honor, self-respect, and self-care are different than the honor, respect, and care others show us. Yes, we are sheep with a herd instinct, but we must choose to follow Jesus and no one else—He is the one we must look up to. We must choose to honor, respect, and care for ourselves because no one else can do that for us (we must love ourselves); not even Jesus can take our place as it is something we must do ourselves with His grace. We choose to believe in ourselves because we are loved by God and are His workmanship. We can't demand respect from others; they can give us respect or deny it, but our self-esteem is in our own hands, and it comes from God loving and believing in us together with loving and believing in ourselves. We must choose to not be needy. A conceited person acts like a parasite in relationships and uses people more than they love them.

There is a relationship between self-pity, conceit, and restorative justice (not retribution or revenge) that I discovered in my interior life. I encountered it one morning, when I realized that I wanted foremost to be respected by another person rather than speak the truth to them in love. If I were to confront the person, the possibility of unsettling the person—and so rob myself of the honor, respect, and esteem I felt in his eyes—did not look appealing. In not speaking up I was trying to protect my honor, but I hated it because I felt an injustice was visited on me that needed to be rectified. I was caught between justice and unhealthy honor. It was a dead end if I chose unhealthy honor above the need for justice because then I'd just endlessly experience self-pity. If I chose justice over unhealthy honor, then the conceit would be struck a blow. I did do this, but if that was all I did, then my conceit would have continued to bother me fiercely. I realized that two further things need to happen for closure:

1. Confessing and repenting of the conceit (selfishness, pride, and fears) I had yet not dealt with in this context, in prayer to God; this would also deal a death blow to my self-pity.
2. After I stood up for the desired justice, when the old conceit tried to reassert itself I needed to choose and commit to justice, instead of unhealthy honor, to cement the victory.

Seeking restorative justice (or stopping injustices, and not seeking retribution or revenge) establishes humility and kills conceit. Growing in gentleness and appreciating the worth of others is important; we do this by caring for others and living out the Golden Rule when it comes to receiving and giving grace. Believing that others have worth gives us faith that we have worth too—they go together. This also helps to kill our conceit, and it turns us into servants instead of pursuing selfish ambition. Fighting off self-pity in this context is also important.

Our battles with conceit cannot be defeated when we refuse people justice because we are too busy protecting our respectability. We have to process our conceitedness in prayer and make the necessary amends. Conceit has crept up in many nooks and crannies in my interior life; it tries to prevent me from forgiving people when my honor is attacked. Acknowledging the conceit, confessing it, repenting in prayer, and renewing my thoughts and beliefs—it all helps me to forgive people much more easily.

6.10: Healing Conceit More Deeply

I see hurt, lies, fears, and conceit as being linked in a Sin-Conduit Structure. Here is a self-explanatory prayer that healed it in my heart and mind:

> "Lord Jesus, I confess that I have a conceit that strongly influences my relating style. I seek praise and admiration from others instead of healthy respect. Who am I kidding? Lord, I confess my conceit as wrong, weak, foolish, sick, and sinful. I regret submitting to it because it is fear driven. I confess that I want to whitewash my exterior and pretend that everything is okay when it is not; that amounts to wearing masks out of fear and weakness. I give up this weak, pathetic, conceited strategy with your help and instead choose to be strong in you, Jesus."

And what are the lies underneath this burden of fear that fuel my conceit?

1. That I'll be rejected if I stand up for the truth.
2. That rejection hurts too much and so must be avoided at all costs.
3. That looking good is more important than standing up for the truth.

> "Lord, I confess that I have given into these fears for most of my life. I regret doing this and I admit that my cowardice is wrong. I have ignored your offer to build up my identity in your unconditional love that leads to the freedom to love others.

> I commit myself to standing up with the truth, as truth is my friend even when people reject me. I give up, with your help Lord Jesus, fearing rejection and caving into it. I also give up, in faith and with your help Jesus, being committed to a false self-image in my makeup. I'm sorry for sinning in these ways. Please forgive and heal me Lord God. Thank you for forgiving me and, I receive this in faith both intellectually and emotionally.

Yes, rejection hurts when it happens. But God's unconditional love conquers; so I believe in His unconditional love which is known as His grace.

> Lord God, I just remembered when I had been rejected as a child at school in South Africa

for lying. I felt again the hurt, the emotions, and the pain as I walked away from that scene. But I was also able to connect with my conceit. There and then you healed me from my conceit, fear, lies, and hurt. Thank you.

Lord God, I'm sorry for being strongly committed to the praise of men so often rather than respecting you as my friend. You are fully deserving of all praise, glory, and worship. Thank you for forgiving me Lord God. Amen.

7 Diagnosing & Healing My Pride

Pride is the next building block in "the tree of knowledge of good and evil" after fear. Pride decides it is superior to all and knows better than anyone else how to approach life and navigate fears—especially in the face of traumatic hurtful experiences. As pride grows so does the tree structure within us. But having pride does not mean we don't have some humility elsewhere in our lives; it is not an all or nothing thing. There are different degrees of pride and humility, and we can grow or shrink in either department.

I know that my pride is alive whether or not I'm aware of it. At its strongest, I recognize it as a powerful dark energy stream within, that is devoid of love. Confronting it with truth helps keep it in check; uncovering the lies around it and replacing them with appropriate truth kills the stronghold, so that my pride becomes manageable in each episode.

People who try to save themselves, by pulling themselves up by their own bootstraps and refusing to humbly call on Jesus, are acting out of pride. They believe lies: that they aren't dependent on God, that He does not care for them, and that He won't help them. Prideful people do not trust anyone and are consumed with fears—hence, possibly wearing masks—and they give themselves all the credit for accomplishments. Pride thinks we are better than other people—hence, the tendency to judge people. When people hurt us, then we can feel justified in our proud reactions or judgments: we take wild jumps in reasoning, we lose our ability to see reality in ourselves and in our relationships, and we see people in distorted ways. This needs to be healed.

People with pride may outright reject God, but many people who are found in churches, synagogues, and mosques on holy days seek power, and so they have pride too; they blindly see God as a way of getting the power they covet. Because pride seeks power to feel in control and to keep fears at bay, it finds its way into our fallen human nature very easily, whether we have religion or not.

To kill the strongholds of pride we need to uncover the lies we believe—in the contexts of the hurts we have experienced and the other unreasonable fears we hold onto. We also need to give up the judgments we make out of our pride. To help humble the pride we need to give God credit for all that He gives to whoever He gives. That means expressing gratitude to God in prayer. Even in the heat of the moment, this requires us to see God with the eyes of faith that say He is good, generous and kind to all. Thanking Him in situations where we feel the opposite is freeing. But this is not enough. We need to confront the pockets of pride we feel that say we are superior and more significant than others, with potent, sober truth, and correct thinking, by inviting Jesus into these spaces to put things into perspective. This requires that we see our pride as foolish and ridiculous, and is one of many things we can do to help renew our minds.

Confessing my foolishness for believing the lies I held onto and confessing the unhealthy history of my proud attitudes is where I started. I then repented in prayer from my proud attitudes, my judgments, and the wrongs and hurts that come from them.

Being open to learning new things, instead of being closed minded, is key to practicing humility. And that means listening to others. But being open is not enough. We need to allow God to teach us, and so we need to pray for humility. To further dethrone pride, we put to death our unreasonable fear by putting our faith in a merciful, caring, graceful, and compassionate Jesus.

Fear motivates us to try to control people, things, and situations that threaten us; this is pride and cowardice saying, "I know better than anyone else." Confessing this to God brings forgiveness, relief, peace, and a sense of starting over. It removes the guilt.

Confession, together with repentance in prayer, renewing the mind, submitting to God, and living out the Golden Rule in the context of grace, helps to deal with our past arrogance: proud habits, proud thinking, proud attitudes, proud judgment, and proud actions. Seeking to do God's will means we don't see ourselves in control and this is very healthy and humble. Spending time with God when we're teachable will slowly help break our pride and move us from negativity to positivity in our journeys.

7.2: Truth Medicines To Overcome Pride

From a website by Fabs[30] we get six medicines to fight off pride: consider the ridiculousness of pride; view each day as an opportunity to forget yourself and serve others; seek a deeper knowledge of God; read biographies of the great saints; remember daily the dangers of pride; and pray for humility. I give a different take on these six medicines, plus I give 15 more of my own:

1. **Consider the ridiculousness of pride.** Pope Francis said, when you believe you are better than others, remember your worst sins and know that you wouldn't wish others to see or know about them.

2. **View each day as an opportunity to forget yourself and serve others.** Consider others as more significant than yourself. This begins at home, on your commute back and forth from work, at work, as well as in your social circles. It starts by rejecting lazy superiority and then grow by seeing the value of people other than oneself (See point 15 below for more).

3. **Seek a deeper knowledge of God.** This is done by pursuing intimacy with God. This requires

---

[30] Cf. www.fabsharford.com, used with permission

becoming dependent on and open with God, not being only sin focused all the time which would keep our focus away from God, which is not wise. We should also meditate on the cross of Jesus and His solidarity with us in the Gospels; this takes away the pressure to improve and the comparisons we make that lead to pride. Read helpful books on prayer, humility, and love that inspire us to follow God and grow in tolerance.

4. **Read the biographies of great saints.** We should also listen to what others say, think, believe and do, without wanting to judge them. This helps us learn from others and is helpful in nurturing humility that leads to love. Everyone is a vehicle of meaning from one degree to another so don't discount anyone's opinion based on religion, color, age, or culture.

5. **Remember daily the danger of pride.** If we find ourselves struggling with pride because we have incorporated a new belief into our paradigm, it does not mean that the belief should be rejected. Often there are other beliefs, ideas, and understandings that need to be incorporated into our lives that will help stabilize us, humble us, and fight off pride. We are complex creatures and we need to realize that much is hidden from us. Patience is required when we come to reject or accept beliefs. Remember that unhealthy independence (from God), when it comes to how we choose to live our lives, is not wise. Pursue real wisdom, that which comes from God when we are living in the moment, and realize that it is practiced and is not just a cursory familiarity with certain concepts or morality.

6. **Pray for help to practice humility.** Why pray for it? Is it because you want to be holy? What is holiness anyways? Holiness is spiritual healthiness, not superficiality, a projected image, or merely a reputation that has no trusted foundations. Praying to be humbled is not necessarily the same as asking for help to practice humility. The former may mean pain and suffering are involved, whereas the latter is more about learning new healthier attitudes.

Note: These next fifteen medicines I came across in my journey; the first four were given to me by the Holy Spirit and have been very helpful in killing my stronghold of pride. Tip 10 was given to me by a friend and has the power to get us to live in the moment; pride and negativity all too often focuses on what is not, whereas humility focuses on what is.

7. **Change your attitude from "impress me" to "I care for you."** This is done by confessing to God, in the moment, the unhealthy attitude of "impress me" and deliberately replacing it with "I care for you" in each context. I have often said to myself in my head, "I don't care…. (about this or that thing)," and I realized there can at times be an unwholesome judgment behind it when I invoke it. I realized that pride, fear, and trust issues between me and my God, needs to be dealt with.

8. **Confess in prayer the exact nature and history of your pride-based attitudes.** Own them as

your own, tell God you're sorry, and asking Him to forgive you while you're still connected to the attitudes you want gone. Scoffing, ridiculing, and thinking the worst of others go against humility and love; repent in prayer from them, and replace the negativity with thanksgiving.

An anally-proud attitude can say, "Impress me; You aren't putting out; I'm better than what you have to offer; I'd rather indulge in my negative, self-pitying, unhappiness because you disappoint me and don't give me the attention I need or want; I have seen better; You have nothing that would make me happy because it takes a lot to impress me; You aren't coming through because you are not creative enough, sacrificial enough, good-looking enough, rich enough, funny enough, kind enough, or special enough, etc. You need to start where you're at. Praying, as suggested in this book won't work if you're not connecting to the attitudes of scoffing, ridiculing, and thinking the worst of others you have entertained.

You need to pray and ask in faith that these dark vices are broken and are replaced by healthy truths. The best way to do so is to stand on God's promises, be conscious and connected to your emotions, desires, commitments, and beliefs, and seek God with all your heart and mind. Ask for the ability to love people more deeply and to not give up searching for what you ask for. Completely killing the dark stream of pride within us can be done with prayer and the right truths. Truth sets us free to love and not judge.

9. **Practice genuine thanksgiving for the good and the bad; the good because it is good and the bad because God can and often does use it for good eventually.** Commit in prayer that God is *absolutely* good: praise Him for His goodness, rest in His love, and focus on Him —not on how holy, pious, and wise you are (in worship, or in your theology, or actions). Worshipping God kills our pride. Worshipping God regularly with Him being the focus is healthy. God does not need our worship; but He ought to be the focus of our worship and praise because that puts the credit for good things in the right place.

Coming into God's presence with thanksgiving, on the holy ground set aside in my heart, is the only way to gain access to God's presence in friendship. I can't cast out Satan with Satan. I can't cast out darkness with darkness. I can't cast out meanness with meanness. I can't cast out hostility with hostility. But when I come with clean energy—a hunger, a thirst, and tears for righteousness—open to being taught, God will grant His grace.

Put your trust in Jesus to save you from your sin, and to help you love supernaturally in your own unique way. Submitting to God also means putting up with negative things that God allows into our lives without complaining, criticizing, or judging (i.e. tolerate the uncomfortable or agree to live with the consequences of other people's hurtfulness towards us and forgive them from the heart). Submitting to God also means submitting to His leadership and teaching—the most authoritative teaching being found in the NT— and then going and doing the good works

God has prepared in advance for me to do.

10. **"Focus on the opportunity in the difficulty; not on the difficulty of the opportunity."** I got this from a friend and it is a fitting way to kill negativity, blaming, and ugly anger, but it can't function in the presence of self-pity. It also helps to kill compulsive-laziness, jealousy, and judging. And it creates a great work ethic and aids the creative process.

This is a principle—that when practiced—allows us to live in the moment. I find that problems and difficulties require processes to diagnose and solve, and when there are no immediate solutions then powerlessness, depression, and self-pity can take over. This can fuel my negativity and anger, and direct my attention away from what I can do. When engaged in a project, I can focus on what is still not done or I can focus on what I am doing and has been done. The former will weigh on me for a long time: stealing my motivation, making me feel a lot of self-pity, and tempting me to give into compulsive-laziness and quit; the latter gets me to live in the moment and makes me feel good.

11. **Start seeing people as special in a true and healthy way**. I used to have these thoughts that had a dark insensitive energy behind it: "Some people *really* think they are, "so damned" special. You just can't trust them. They are so predictable. They will do anything to pull one over on you. They only care for themselves. I see through them. They think they are oh so special. They think they own the world. I'm better than them."

These thoughts came when I had been hurt badly. I was a scoffer; skeptical, sour, jaded, and had no hope in people. These words drip with self-pity, pride, jealousy, hurt, and an "I will show them I'm better and more special" attitude.

People who have been hurt badly can lash out in this way; their hurting ends up hurting others. But this does not have to be permanent. Forgiveness directed towards your enemies will bring healing, and renewal of your mind. Using "I" statements (instead of judging people like in the rant above) will restore one to sanity. This gets you in touch with your nobler attitudes, healthier energy, and feelings God has put in your hearts.

I can see how irrational the thoughts are behind some of my attitudes or feelings. When I feel a carnal insensitivity within myself and think the lie; "I'm better than them," I need to counter it with, "I'm not better than them; we are what we are." This is the medicine that helps to cure the rise of pride (and contempt) within us. These truths need to be used to confront the dark energy of pride. Shallowness won't achieve anything; we need to go deeper and deeper to get to the foundation of the tree structure within us. We have power to choose our thoughts, words, tone of voice, and the energy of the words, so that our relating style can be healing and restorative instead of toxic. People respond to kindness more warmly than anger.

If we don't see that each person bears the image of God stamped on their souls, then we will have an arrogance within us that will peep out every now and then trying to flaunt our superiority. We need to respect the whole person. After I have prayed through my strongholds of arrogance, I then counter my pride with the truth saying, "All of us are special in our own unique ways," together with praying out loud that my walls of superiority are dismantled through trust in Jesus. I forgive my enemies, pledging to care and love them. And I declare all real estate in my heart to belong to God, and no longer to the devil. God has filled my heart with good things and has also helped me to love outwardly in more intimate ways, which means I am more victorious against pride through Jesus' care, grace, truth and mercy.

Many times, praying in a deeper way about a sinful stronghold is needed. Here are two such ways:

a) **Praying the scriptures.** Here is an example of my own from the Gospels: After Jesus taught the Sermon on the Mount that was all about humility in action, a leper comes up to Him and says that if Jesus is willing He can heal him. Jesus does. To pray this, I visualize myself as the leper (with an attitude of pride in my life being my skin disease) I kneel before Jesus and ask Him to heal me. And He does.

b) **Asking Jesus to heal memories.** Going back to our painful memories, looking for where Jesus is in those hurtful scenes, and asking Him to speak healing into the painful memory can bring health too (there are many healthy books on this topic). He might speak a word to us that opens up an overlooked area of sin: or that we need to deal with in prayer, that can possibly resolve our painful memory, or so that it no longer triggers sinful responses in our relationships.

12. **Use my higher rights to sacrifice my lower rights.** Pride says we need to have the best, be the best, or have what others have. Pride often means an attitude of self-entitlement (i.e. selfishness). With such attitudes anger is not far away when what we have is threatened, violated, ridiculed, stolen or disrespected. The way to conquer this struggle is to deal with the "tree of knowledge of good and evil" within and then the "sin nature" through prayer. This is done by dealing with self-pity and anger (and the pressure we put on ourselves) and not to minimize the wrongs done to us. We also need to refrain from judging people in order to love them to the end.

In practice, the way to navigate situations where our rights are trampled on or violated is to not minimize the infractions, and to give up our judgments. Because if we minimize the wrongs, then we are moving personal boundaries, which goes against the principles of justice and respect. When we minimize infractions and judge the flesh screams self-pity, anger, or both. The reason we deal with the "sin nature" in prayer is because we don't want to react in an ugly or sinful way towards any person. But if we refuse to minimize the wrongs people do to us and give up judgments, then we can stand up for ourselves in respectful ways with healthy self-esteem just like Jesus did.[31] This is different than having an attitude of self-entitlement or being selfish. If we refuse to minimize wrongs and judge, then we won't be as susceptible to self-pity or beating ourselves up, and it will be easier to give up those rights in the name of love and peace while not acting like doormats. This is what Saint Paul also alluded to in his first letter to the Corinthians.[32]

Everything we have is a gift from God. Even if we fought to keep the devil from stealing it and if we do own it, then we can freely give it up in the right situations with the right energy—if we are not selfish, not judgmental and don't try to minimize the loss. We can't demand it from God even if it is a "right" or a "normal" part of everyday human existence. Self-made people think everyone—including God— owes them what they hold dear; they refuse to give it up under any circumstances and will fight tooth and nail to keep it. Selfish and judgmental people find it hard to give up anything for other people.

But people who respect God also have pride, and so can and do have varying degrees of entitlement (i.e. selfishness): dearly held onto rights, things we hold onto that we feel very strongly about, and sometimes things we protect in very mean judgmental ways. When our rights are violated we will get angry. If we indulge in self-pity (rooted in selfishness and conceit), then we will not be kind and full of love for our enemies after they have violated us. When we deal healthily with our self-pity in prayer, then we will love our enemies more like Jesus does. We will also give up judgments and forgive more easily.

But we can't do this through our own strength, wisdom, and self-righteousness. We need to approach this task through humble prayer, take Jesus as our model, and use Scripture as our encouragement and support. When we handle the negative in a positive way, then this is healthy; gentleness and meekness will result, and my enemies will notice that something is different.

When we have difficulty in forgiving a coworker: for not respecting us; for not obeying a rule that in our eyes symbolizes respect for us when kept; or for making us go farther than our honor permits, then the anger can only be eliminated when we give up our rushing displays to protect our honor and give up our right to the respect we covet or desire from others. This is done by dismantling all Sin-Conduit Structures in my personal "tree of knowledge of good and evil," as

---

[31] Cf. John 18:22
[32] Cf. 1 Corinthians 6:7

outlined in this book.

In prayer, I have found confessing and repenting from holding onto entitlements in a rude, mean, and jerk-like manner is just as important as dealing with the roots to these in "the tree of knowledge of good and evil" within me. It is so easy to think that people owe me, and to treat them with respect only so long as they serve a purpose in my life. If I am humble I will be able to love people not because of what their power, intellect, and creativity can do for me, but because they have worth, dignity, and a purpose of their own.

For example, I have strongly felt entitled to a quietness so that I could determine my own thoughts: to not let others determine the direction of my thoughts, and to not be pestered with annoying sounds. When I did not get the quiet I wanted, I'd go to a nasty and self-pitying place inside of me and when pushed to it I'd act like a jerk. I struggled for years trying to wrestle this issue to the ground and find peace. It was a learning curve for me. At first, temporary measures were learned to keep me from acting like a control freak or jerk. Then I slowly went deeper with Jesus to places where I understood how pride, judgments, self-pity, anger, pressure, minimization, jealousy, selfishness, meanness, and an "eye for an eye" mentality were responsible for my lack of tolerance. Dismantling the Sin-Conduit Structures in my life that contained these energized commitments was key to finding victory in this area.

13. **Practice forgiveness and process my emotions in healthy ways.** Not forgiving others punishes me—not those who hurt me. Also, I need to deal with my anger, confusion, and broken expectations when they show up overriding my feelings in prayer to God. I need to renew my mind with His responses and with the help of "I" statements that move me from judging people to telling the truth.

Knowing that God understands my struggles and getting in touch with my feelings goes a long way to healthily processing them. Not processing my emotions, limits or snuffs out my ability to practice the Golden Rule. In processing my feelings, I get in touch with how God has wired me to be noble, kind, pure, healthy, and at peace. The "flesh" can't compete with the Holy Spirit—for whom I am made.

14. **Practice humility; not just dismantling the stronghold of pride:** Yes, there is a place for dismantling the stronghold of pride, but something must take its place. There is death, but it is not completed without resurrection. Jesus is the Resurrection. Committing to viewing myself the way God sees me is a part of humility. This isn't supposed to be a static state, but a dynamic one and a work in progress.

Let's not settle for following the letter of the law: having to have things personally fair all the time, demanding our rights, being first all the time, and only being concerned about getting to heaven. "Whoever tries to save his life will lose it; but whoever loses his life will preserve it."[33] Jesus' commands are high enough to steer us in the right direction, and He comes to us not only to help us fulfill the OT law through keeping the higher law of love. He taught us the Sermon on the Mount so that we care for our neighbors in tangible ways. When we grow in the fruit of the Spirit then we know that we are growing in humility.

The strategy to confront negative strongholds is to admit they are in our lives, and to say to them, "I don't need you right now. I give you up with Jesus' help through faith, because God provides for my needs with His grace and peace." Grace is the Holy Spirit's empowering presence. We commit our sins because we come to falsely believe that they will fulfill our wants and needs. Admitting this, mourning the losses incurred by the sins because they *really* promise emptiness, and committing to and connecting with Jesus as Prince of Peace are all important in moving on to healthier pastures. I need to do this emotionally as well as intellectually. In this way, I count as dead previous strongholds of sin, and embrace the full life promised by Jesus. I turn to the Holy Spirit to overcome my sin.

Nature hates vacuums so I should replace my sin energy with virtues (i.e. grace). Grace comes from the peace and the presence of God. The process of repenting prayer asks me to deal with the lies that I believed when I became a slave to certain sins that became strongholds in my life. These lies are the reasons why certain idols were used to try to satisfy my needs.

For instance, if I was hurt by being rejected, I can be deceived into believing the lie that being conceited will protect my self-image and give me the sense that I am still likable. Or, I might believe the lie that I need to project a strong and arrogant attitude to others so they won't think I am hurt and weak inside. Both these strategies help to destroy the image of God in which I am made. They destroy healthy identity; they rob me of being fully loved and reciprocating love.

Overnight success won't necessarily happen, but a gradual process of renewal will be formed as new patterns of thinking, talking, and acting are slowly built. The "thou shalt not" or the "no, no, no" by themselves in the face of carnal energy are not sufficient for positive victory and healthy change; they leave us stuck and defeated. We need negative attitudes and habits to be replaced with positive attitudes and actions. Jesus offers this to all of us through His presence, His teaching, His commands, and His guiding strength—all correctly focused.

15. **Humility grows when I aim for love.** Humility does not grow when our foremost aim is to only acquire truth, because all we are looking for then are informative insights that may broaden our knowledge (which can lead to pride). And we won't get beyond "truth" to connecting with people—which is what love is all about. When I am people focused, then in

---

[33] Luke 17:33

caring for them I will find ways to grow in love, which means growing in humility too.

16. **Focus on whatever is true, positive, uplifting, kind, and gentle.** The ability to love is sustained by focusing on trusting Jesus and nurturing clean and pure energy within to love people. Once I have dealt with a disappointment, I focus on Jesus and doing His will. I refuse to let my negative emotions guide me relationally, because if I do, then they will reinforce my self-pity and people won't like being around me. Jesus is Lord, and He has authority, but He is gentle, kind, and honest. He does not cruelly and angrily force me into obedience. So I too should not unkindly and irately expect obedience from myself and others. It is God's kindness that leads me to repentance.

17. **Become able to accept people's choices when they say no.** This opens doors of love in our hearts, makes us generous, kind, and compassionate instead of rigid, mean, judgmental, and angry all the time.

18. **When we get healthier in an area within, we ought not compare ourselves to others.** Because then we undo the blessings coming from God. We reveal this pride by giving off the attitude "I'm good, intelligent, and better than them," vs. "they're bad, stupid, and worse than me." And we realize that the line between good and evil goes through our hearts, not in between people, groups, cultures, and traditions. We need to give up this belief wherever it is hidden within our hearts and minds regarding all our relationships.

19. **When we get proud of the little humility we do have, then healing comes when we confess it to God, repent from it in prayer, renew our minds, submit to God, and accept our crosses.**

20. **When we start to spout off about how we have achieved, earned, or created things through our own pain, choices, work, studies, or intellect, then we need to humble ourselves and admit to God's part in our processes.**

21. **Embrace God's truth, grace, and presence found in Jesus. Jesus will never leave you nor forsake you.**

7.3: Diagnosing And Healing Pressure And Force

Humility is gentle, whereas pride uses pressure (usually focused inwardly on ourselves and manipulatively on others) and force (which is usually directed outwards at others). Pressure hardens our hearts and violates other people's boundaries; it is often angry, abusive, cold, hateful, mean, and sinister. Pressure uses a whip to get its stinging way usually with the aim of misguided perfectionism. When pride uses force, it does so because it treats people as objects or tools to be picked up or dropped when needed.

There is little peace in the hearts of those who put pressure on themselves through pride. There is little community for those who hold fearlessly and insensitively to using force to get their way. People with these characteristics will treat animals and people the same way—poorly. Using force is usually very ugly.

The only way to stop using pressure and force on ourselves and others is to confess these sins to God, repent in prayer, and then deal with them in the context of our hurts, fears, and pride. We need to discover how to see people and animals in a healthy way, which means truths need to uproot the relational lies we have believed. People with this dynamic operating in their lives, need to learn to see the humanity in others and within themselves. They have believed lies about themselves usually in the context of rejections or having been hurt by others. Healing of memories through prayer can *really* help in such situations.

When grace flows through me it is the surest way to help me stop applying pressure, force, and manipulation on others and myself through using anger, self-pity, and guilt.

7.4: Diagnosing And Healing Arrogance

Arrogance is defined as an offensive display of superiority or self-importance. It can be a smile on the face when tears are more appropriate. It is the most hurtful and hostile kind of pride. When we think we are better than others (i.e. more special or superior) we will be tempted to go out of our way to rub our supposed superiority in the faces of those people we despise. Usually the arrogant are hurting people, wounded or numbed from the pain within. Usually a hurt person will end up hurting others. Arrogance goes out of its way to hurt people and is devoid of love because of this.

Arrogance means we are hungry for grace, but have not found grace because of pride, unbelief, lies, unconfessed sin, hurt, or resentments. Arrogance is an attitude that says I don't care about other people. It says my interests are most important, and it searches and applies itself to getting what it wants. But when something blocks its way or when people block the completion of a goal from an arrogant person, they will either exude meanness, self-pity, or both. The meanness will be directed at others, whereas self-pity can be a sign of defeat and anger turned inwards. Arrogance says I only care about myself, and my goals are more important than others.

If we don't care about people when horrible situations occur, then we can't love those people involved. Not caring comes from pride. So, giving up our pride will lead the way to humility and caring more deeply for others as time goes by.

There is no blanketed prayer that will remove our not caring all at once. To care more for people on our journey, we need to give up the attitude that we and our concerns are the most important, and that we are the center of the universe. More than that, we need to acknowledge that God is the center of the universe in all of the places where we are uncaring about people, from the past up to the present. But we shouldn't hit ourselves over the head with truth. We have to believe in ourselves and be strong in healthy ways.

Present uncomfortable circumstances can be triggered by unprocessed uncaring attitudes from the past. These uncomfortable moments are doorways we can walk through to caring more deeply for others, and we can do so with strategic prayer, liberating truths, and Jesus' help.

Anger, pressure, and conceit also need to be dealt with to move from not caring for others to being compassionate towards them. The way out for us not caring for others comes from replacing lies with truth that liberates us. It has been said that if I look for truth to love I won't necessarily end up loving, because as time goes by concepts, ideas, and principles may become more important than love. Also, if I seek power to love, I won't necessarily love either because I may always be waiting for more power to love. And when I'm weak I may not love because I complain that I don't have enough power to love. Focusing on love *out of caring* leads to the ability to love. Love is the way—not concepts, not power, but love. Love grows in weakness and not in strength. Putting concepts or power first distracts me from love. Truth is important only as far as aiding me in love. Ultimately, the ability or grace to love comes from God, whether I am weak or strong.

Ministry is not about holding onto power, position, and pedigree so I can somehow love and speak truth authoritatively. I must focus on love; doing to others what I would want done to me in the context of grace. In this way, I will live out my destiny and overcome the lies and obstacles in the way of love being able to flow.

As a Christian, I trust in Jesus to save me from my sins and to help me to love meaningfully. To renew my mind, I need to unpack the judgmental boxes I put people into, and see people as special in the kindest ways possible. Satan sows the lie in my mind that others are proud saying, "They think they are something special when they are not. I'm the humble one—not them." And when I believe this I end up judging others and being more proud and arrogant than those I have judged. The reason this lie is so powerful is that it is done in the context of being hurt by others. In the past, when I was hurt by others, I ended up having a jaded view of people and started having a crisis of identity—fertile ground for fallen angels to grow arrogance and hardness of heart in a person's life.

After I thoroughly prayed through these issues, I willingly began to lower my "walls" to let go of my arrogance, and recommit to love and intimacy. This allowed more wholesome thought processes to take root, and enabled me to slowly let go of those thought processes generated by the pain body within formed by those hurts received from others. I became more conscientious about owning these painful memories and the attitudes they generated which helped me in the process of releasing them. "The tree of knowledge of good and evil" is intact, alive, and at work in whomever it has taken root in. The mind may be unaware, but the dark energy streams of pride in the tree are active whether we're aware of them or not.

8 Diagnosing & Healing The Selfish-Love Branches Of The Tree Of Knowledge Of Good And Evil In Me

Selfish-love is one of two building blocks that spring from pride (the other is coveting). The building block of selfish-love is found on the left side of "the tree of knowledge of good and evil." It looks like love, but it is not based on truth, honesty, or healthiness.

Abandoning love often gets initiated out of self-pity, when people jettison their relationship with God because of some grievance; they decide to live life on their own terms, seeking to make themselves happy through their own means or initiative.

Selfish-love uses people and things to optimize pleasure, and likes to discard them when not needed. Selfish-love kills real love. It cares only for itself.

If I try to push people with needs and requests out of my way, then I am giving in to an uncaring nature. I should not try to force things to my liking exteriorly just like it is unhealthy to do it interiorly through pressure. I can do my best to fit people into my life or I can choose to put myself and my pleasure first. Let selfish-love die, and care for people more. Selfish-love seeks to feel good at the expense of people and will use people for pleasure alone.

When I get restless, impatient, angry, and self-pitying then my selfish-love comes to life. I won't be a Good Samaritan when I abandon love. The following will help to kill this aspect of uncaring: finding out where I am at and confessing these things to God; repenting in prayer; and submitting to God out of the renewing of my mind.

In order to find healing, I must also pray through and process my related pride and fear; how they relate to my broken relationship with God and my broken relationships with people I have conflict with. Then, I can focus on living in the moment instead of demanding that everything be made over to suit me. Selfishness and uncaring attitudes promise me happiness, but they never console me. It is a nightmare in the making.

Selfish-love also desires to feel good at the expense of health. It leads to compulsive-laziness and compulsive-indulging, but is cured through the grace that comes through prayer and changing what I value.

The more I remove my own idols from my God-shaped vacuum within, in prayer (inviting Jesus to take His rightful places in my heart) and renewing my mind with healthy truth and thinking, (ridding myself of angry pressure and self-pity as a means to getting my own way,) then the more it will make practicing self-discipline and self-control realistic (one will know perhaps for the first time that it is doable with God's empowering presence). Putting angry pressure on myself kills self-control. And fear creates impatience.

As for the thinking part, I need to decide not to go after stuff only because it tastes good, it feels good, or it is an easier lazy way. If certain feelings lead to healthiness — good — if not, then one puts those feelings to death by changing how one thinks and believes through prayer. One needs to commit to living for a higher purpose than pleasure alone to heal selfish-love. So how does one get started?

In feeling our selfish-love emotions, we will get to explore and know the thinking and rationale behind them. This will then help us to counter corrupt thoughts and beliefs, by exploring healthy and holy thoughts (whose inspiration is the Holy Spirit), and choosing health over feeling instant gratification alone. I need to consciously put my faith in Jesus to save me from my sins regularly. Then I submit to God; and resist the devil. Death without resurrection is incomplete; killing the stronghold of selfish-love is empty without focusing on healthy love, and accepting God's will in the uncomfortable situations in my life.

Tackling Selfish-love in My Life

I had the following attitude in me where God took the initiative to bring me healing. It was a difficult challenge where I felt things to be so intolerable and unfair. I found myself needing encouragement from many sources, as the wickedness of my selfish-love was laid bare within me. The Sin-Conduit Structure took this form:

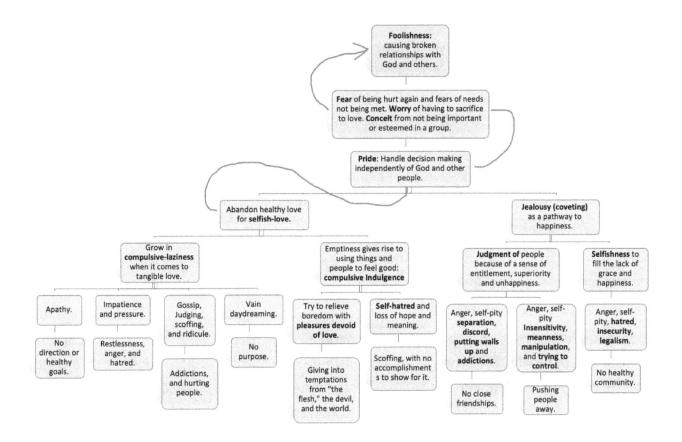

The Situation

I had a dark energy within me where I compulsively and mechanically fitted people, events, and circumstances into my schedule only caring that they served my wants and needs (it is horrible I know). I basically used both people and situations to serve my own selfish desires. Because of this I was a toy of the devil whenever this dynamic operated within me. I struggled to be free of it. This energy within me was petty, anal, legalistic, and caring only for my own desires and pleasures. I did not think about praying about it until God put His finger on it.

Prayer

Lord God, with your help through faith, I give up this dynamic of selfish-love in my life—of caring for others only to the degree that they served my interests. I have a long history of doing this, especially as my schizophrenia progressed and happy moments were hard to come by. With your help Lord Jesus, I give up my demands that others fit into my schedule. I give up my impatience, restlessness, self-pity, anger, hatred, and uncaring attitudes towards the people in my life. I admit I wanted all of this because I had an inflated sense of self-worth and pride, and I felt my happiness to be more important than others; and I give this up, with your help, Lord Jesus Christ. I confess all this sin to You, the Living God, and receive your forgiveness and healing both intellectually and emotionally. Thank you, Lord Jesus!

Going Deeper in Prayer

Lord Jesus, I confess my selfish-love of using people, and believing the lie that people have no real immediate worth. Please forgive me this horribleness. Lord, I surrender my commitments to using people; with your help, I give up using people for my own selfish ends! Thank you! The truth is people have infinite worth in Your eyes, and I choose to agree with you, the Living God, in this matter.

Lord Jesus, I confess my pride in thinking I alone have worth. Through your grace, I reject the lie that I alone have worth; I give up this belief with your help.

I confess my fears of losing out, of being forgotten, of not being happy, of going home empty-handed, and of missing out on things other people take for granted. Lord Jesus, I give up these fears, expectations, and beliefs and put my trust in you the real Shepherd who cares for me, and loves me! Thanks for promising to do just that!

Lord Jesus, I confess my history of not trusting people — my parents, and loved ones. I confess not trusting you the Almighty God more fully. I give up my sourness, and my despair, and need to control things through anger and self-pity all the time. Thank you so much for loving me and forgiving me these things, Jesus! Thank you for coming alongside me and imparting your peace, grace, and presence so I know I'm not alone and can face my challenges head-on. Amen!

Fruits

The desperate, dark, mechanical type of energy went away. Temporarily, the heightened impatience, restlessness, anger, and hatred were gone, but I would have to go deeper to be rid of my impatience. I started connecting with people and being touched by them more; and I found them interesting instead of just wanting to use them.

The selfish-love in this situation had also caused compulsive-indulging, and a measure of self-control was returned to me in this area also.

Going Even Deeper

Later, God put His finger on my impatience; I realized that I struggled with anger when I was impatient. And then God showed me that I also had hatred in my heart because I saw others as inconvenient—and I hated it. I was then led in prayer to give up my anger and hatred in the many different contexts where my impatience arose. Hence, the Sin-Conduit Structure:

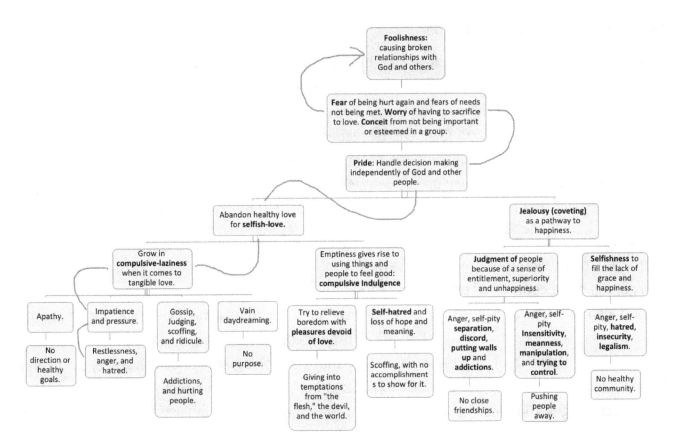

Going Deeper And Dealing With More Selfish-love

Lord God, I suffer from being impatient with others. Getting on the bus has become a circus; people pushing and jostling for position to get the best seats. I have participated in this by coveting a good seat above showing warmth towards my fellow bus passengers. This comes out of my compulsive-laziness. I didn't want to love if it would cost me something (like giving up a comfortable seat). I have selfish-love here too: I pushed people, blocked people, and established my presence in an unhealthy way. I attempted to get better positions or prized seats—saying no to love. My pride is alive saying, "My needs, and my wants come first," and "I come first and I'm the center of the universe". This is motivated by my fears of having to suffer while loving and of having to give up some comfort. Lord, I give these fears and sins all up, with your help through faith in you, Jesus. Lord, I also admit that this is rooted in my own foolishness. I was hard on myself in South Africa. I was rejected by peers as a child for lying, so I berated myself for my failures on the playground. Lord, I have been hard on myself, and therefore I have been nasty towards others too. I forgive my peers for being so hard on me. Lord God, please forgive me my sins in this context. I regret sinning. I'm sorry for these sins, and I give them up with your help in faith, Lord Jesus. Thank you for forgiving and promising to heal me. Amen!

Note: There is nothing wrong with competing for a seat on a bus in a warm, kindly manner; but I need to do so in healthy and respectful ways, and to give up my seat for those more in need.

Many Times We Need To Go Deeper

If the strongholds of selfish-love described in this section do not completely go away after fighting it in this manner, then we have to go deeper. We have to think about healing our spirits: by forgiving the agents of our past hurts and ourselves in related contexts; by giving up judgments and attacks towards God; and by recommitting to receive God's grace and to give that grace back to the people in our lives. Moreover, there is the work of renewing our minds, with Jesus' help, in prayer; giving up the way we wrongly view people, and giving up using anger and self-pity to get our way. When this is all accomplished, then there is real freedom.

I need to remind myself that doing things that require effort will not always become easy, and that I can't coast by through life if I am serious about doing God's will. Going by my feelings (to feel good), in the contexts of overcoming compulsive-indulging and compulsive-laziness, is never a good idea; it makes living life fully, practicing self-control, doing acts of love, and caring about working, almost impossible. If I do abandon effort, initiative and caring, I will become useless, and self-control will never be a reality. Coasting and abandoning effort nullifies grace, truth, and the prayers and strategies found in this book. Coasting and abandoning effort means we are living according to the "flesh" or the "sin nature" and they waste or block the supply of Jesus' grace.

Having successfully found freedom from the stronghold of selfish-love, it must be said that temptations to selfish-love are normal because the "sin nature" does not go away in this life. What we can expect is to not exaggerate grievances and distort things in conflicts; we deal with setbacks proportionately.

8.2: Diagnosing And Healing Compulsive-Laziness

The stronghold of compulsive-laziness grows out of our selfish-love in "the tree of knowledge of good and evil" within us. Compulsive-laziness only cares about itself and can't love. It has no depth, purpose, or meaning. When we have this sickness of compulsive-laziness we usually bully ourselves to achieve things out of guilt. We don't want to go the extra mile, and get angry when asked to change our plans or do extra stuff. We need to see this as wrong and ask the Holy Spirit for the gift of self-discipline. We start by reasoning with the Holy Spirit to find our bearings. After we are led to confess our compulsive-laziness to God—owning our history of it, saying it is wrong and that we are sorry, and asking for and receiving forgiveness with thanksgiving, from God (not just intellectually but emotionally)—then we repent in prayer from it. We do this to deal with our history of compulsive-laziness. Then we pray about it as it relates to our selfish-love, pride, fear, and broken relationships (foolishness).

When my compulsive-laziness tries to reassert itself again and again I need to confess, and repent in prayer again and again from using anger and pressure to motivate my efforts. We will have to address this in the different circumstances where it is alive in our hearts, but we also need to start thinking about healthier motivations to replace the void of apathy.

As we do this we become open to the Holy Spirit's gift of self-discipline and Jesus' teaching meant to bring about healthy thoughts, beliefs, and actions. We need to submit to God in this area and resist the devil. The restorative medicine is to seek meaning in love. And love is active and based on truth. Personally, I look to my family and place of work to find outlets of meaningful giving.

I never really thought of myself as a servant, and I did not have the attitude and healthy disposition of a servant whose heart is wholly devoted to God. But reflecting on how entitlement operates in my life has brought this more into focus for me. So much written in the Sermon on the Mount is only possible for me when I give up my stranglehold on personal justice and grasping my rights. I must instead follow the example of Jesus with His grace and the Holy Spirit through transformative prayer. My heart and mind embrace and focus on healthier beliefs, motives, and energy and are led by the Holy Spirit through truth. This fruit is from the Holy Spirit through strategic prayer with Jesus' help—not through analysis or psycho-analysis.

Attempting to love like Jesus does by using our own energy leads to a struggle that can't be won and invites plenty of self-pity; it is self-defeating and is impossible unless the sinful strongholds from the past are dealt with through prayer and wisdom. Those who seek to follow and obey Jesus and care about living out the Sermon on the Mount will make great strides in becoming healthy servants in the likeness of Jesus.

Practicing the Golden Rule will get us out of our comfort zone. We do this not by just giving mental assent to the rule, but we imagine what it looks like and set out to do it. We may have blockages to making the Golden Rule practical at times and this calls for patience and perseverance. Unforgiving attitudes, fears, pride, and selfish-love can all be blocks to loving others in caring obedience to Jesus. Getting rid of these blocks is done through the strategies outlined in this book. Living out the Golden Rule is easier when we embrace and accept our crosses: difficult circumstances and people, temptations, and the pull of our "sin nature" with the view of overcoming them through faith, hope, and love.

We will slowly learn to see things differently. Instead of seeing things as burdens and nuisances, we see them as opportunities where we start doing something good with God's help; to contribute instead of acting selfishly in relation to others. This will involve prayers where we join with God in faith to change our attitudes and the way we see and act. Wisdom means that we put to death living by our feelings alone and trust Jesus to save us from our sins instead.

We are made for work, and work is made for us. As the NT Scripture attests: "For we are God's handiwork, created in Christ Jesus to do good works, which God prepared in advance for us to do."[34] All too often the devil tries to steal the good that we can do by stoking our sense of outrage, pride, and fear when we are asked by people to do things that we know we should not have to be asked to do. In turn, we are loaded with feelings of guilt, shame, and low self-esteem. This is not the way it ought to be. If we pursue God's will, confess and repent in prayer, and receive His forgiveness after we fail, then we can overcome compulsive-laziness. The intensity of prayer needs to be proportionate to the sin.

Also, I need to live in the moment if I want to subdue the stronghold of compulsive-laziness. I need to stop indulging in too much daydreaming and useless fantasies. A way to do this is to focus on my opportunities and not the difficulties in the opportunities. This can give me a sense of achievement and healthy pride, and it will help eat away at my low self-esteem and expectations that others should make me happy.

People who dwell on injustices can fall into self-pity, end up having victim mentalities or negative outlooks on life, and draw negative things to themselves. This steals our joy—a fruit of the Spirit. And if joy is a fruit of the Spirit, then self-pity is a malady of the "flesh" which means it is sinful. The only ways to kill it is to not feed it, and pray strategically so that God can cleanse us from it with refreshing truth. And to practice thanksgiving for all that we receive from God and others.

I remember as a young child being summoned to do yard work while my sister and brother got to watch TV. I wept bitterly with great self-pity, screamed unfairness, and hated the labor. Why? I believe there were five reasons dealing with my direction and aim in life at the time:

1. I did not have my father's **values.** What I saw as important was immature, and only mixed with compulsive-laziness and instant self-gratification... not of creating something longer lasting and more enduring and less selfish.
2. I did not have my father's **vision.** I was not able to see the opportunity beckoning me or the ability to see the fruits that my labor could bring.
3. I did not have my father's **desires.** My only reason for doing it was because I had to and not because it would bring beauty and pleasure to others.
4. I did not have my father's **willingness to sacrifice** for something better. He was willing to give up the pleasures of entertainment for the pleasure of accomplishing something worthy of his time and efforts.
5. I did not have my father's healthy **commitment to persevere**. I just wanted to get it over and done with.

To help stop the kind of compulsive-laziness talked about here we might think we only need to pray for healthier values and desires, clearer vision, a willingness to sacrifice, and the grace to

---

[34] Ephesians 2:10

commit to something greater. But as good as this may seem it doesn't go far enough, because we do not take responsibility for our sins and ignore the process of repenting done in prayer. First, in prayer, we need to give up our use of self-pity and anger to get our way and we need to give up our demands that others make us happy. Secondly, we need to repent from our hypocrisy, and our wrongly judging others for their supposed laziness. Thirdly, we need to dismantle our unhealthy values using these steps as a guideline:

1. **Write down our false values when it comes to work (these are the lies we have believed): "_____"** (i.e. not completely caring about the work; thinking my life is more important than loving others through work, just wanting to get it over with; believing work can't be fun; not caring deeply about quality; just filling the allotted quotas; just showing up to collect a paycheck, etc.).

2. **Write down the sins one has committed (because of the false values and lies one believes): "_____"** (i.e. coasting, being lazy, wasting time, pretending to be a hard worker, criticizing coworkers, leaving extra work for coworkers, getting away with the minimum, not taking responsibility when issues arrive, etc.).

3. **Pray something like the following:** Dear Jesus, I confess my sins of "_____" (Step 2) and the lies that I believed that gave life to my false values of "_____" (Step 1). And I give them up with your help in faith. I receive your forgiveness and healing both intellectually and emotionally. Please help me to renew my mind, values, and attitudes so I will have a healthy work ethic. I now choose to live life with your lavish grace and to live my life built on your truth. Lord Jesus, thank you. Amen.

Example: Tackling Compulsive-laziness in My Life

The following lies became a hidden part of my values when I was summoned to do yard work by my father, and they put a big burden of negativity into my attitudes towards work.

1. I believed the lie that work was not fun.
2. I believed the lie that work was not satisfying.
3. I believed the lie that work was boring.

I worked hard most of my life, but it was driven by an angry, mean, pressure I put on myself. It was based on a sense of duty and not love, joy or pleasure; it was without a real peace and consolation in knowing I was doing something meaningful for others besides myself. Praying through these using "the tree of knowledge of good and evil" diagram below was the way to have victory over this stronghold of compulsive-laziness in my life:

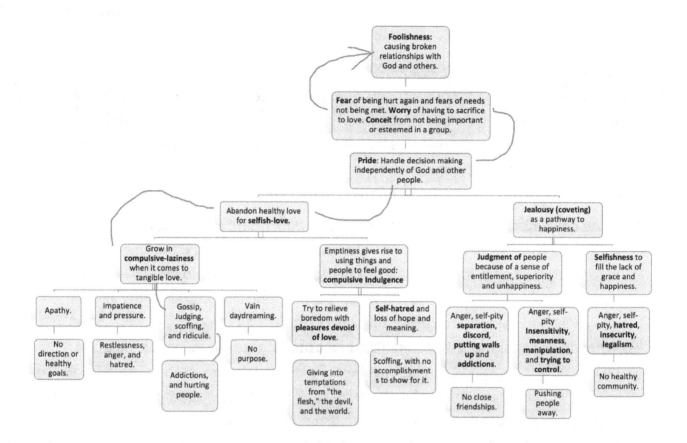

Prayer

"Lord Jesus, I confess that I have approached school and work by believing lies that led to compulsive-laziness most of my life. I give up this compulsive-laziness and choose to give up believing these lies now, with your help through faith. I confess that I consoled myself with the pleasures of compulsive-laziness instead of investing your energy in the aptitudes you gave me. This is selfish-love, and I give this up with your help in faith. Instead of finding meaning and purpose in learning and work, I have put enormous amounts of hatred and pressure on myself to achieve. I confess this as wrong and give up this strategy now, with your help Lord Jesus and through faith in you. I have been motivated by fear and pride, only concerned about how others saw my achievements, instead of loving them through the deeds. I give this up with your help now and embrace your forgiveness and healing now through faith. Thank you, Father God, Lord Jesus, and Holy Spirit. Amen."

A Revelation

I realized that this was not the only principal source of my compulsive-laziness. A short while later something else was triggered. Yes, my working attitude did become healthier, but then an incident occurred where scoffing gushed out of me in the context of work. Someone who I was working with asked me to trade tasks, and I felt insulted and hurt. Self-pity, anger, and ridicule were pouring out of my heart. Thankfully, I hid what was happening within and decided to pray about it thoroughly when I had a chance.

More Prayer

"Lord God, I confess that my heart oozes with scoffing, arrogance, anger, and self-pity in the context of work. When I was asked to trade tasks it triggered this dark energy within me, and I'm sorry for allowing this to grow in my heart all these years. I have disrespected people made in your image thinking my honor, worth, and abilities are better than and more important than other people's abilities, feelings, and worth. I give this all up with your help in faith Lord Jesus, because you are the great physician.

Lord God, please take from me the above vices, and replace them with the virtues of care, connection, and empathy. Thank you for loving me, forgiving me, and healing me. I receive your graces and gifts emotionally as well as intellectually, Lord Jesus. And I choose to become gracious towards those I meet daily out of your strength, because you are my pillar of strength and never leave me to my own devices. Thank you. Amen."

Going Deeper

Repenting in such a way as to restore the compassion that God had originally given and the devil stole from me. To do this consider the following Sin-Conduit Structure and corresponding Sin-Anatomy Table beneath it:

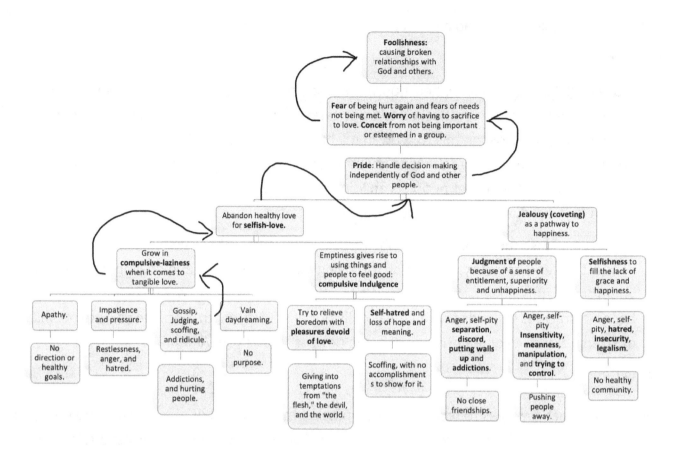

Scoffing	Compulsive laziness	Abandoned Love	Pride	Fear	Foolishness
	<=	<=	<=	<=	<= Cause and Effect
Scoffing at those close to me and those far off. They must all be paid according to my burdens, so that we all suffer together.	I choose to have no mercy on others: I refuse to lift a finger to help others in tight spots.	If I have to suffer, then so must others.	I come first. My well-being is more important than the well-being belonging to others.	Fear that I'll be the only one without the goodies.	If I'm exiled it shouldn't be me alone. I believe life is unfair. Why do I get the short end of the stick all of the time.
Did this for years without realizing a way out…				.	
Confession & Repenting in Faith =>	=>	=>	=>	=>	

Prayer

Lord, I confess that I have lacked real in depth compassion and caring for others most of my life. Please forgive me. [Done Rene] Thanks Jesus! Lord God, I give up this lack of caring loaded with scoffing and hardness with your help through faith in you Lord Jesus.

Lord God, I confess that I registered mostly zeros when it came to the beatitude: "Blessed are the merciful for they will receive mercy." Please forgive me my shallowness. [Done] Thanks Jesus. Lord God, I give up this insensitivity with your help through faith in you. I choose to be merciful from here onwards with your grace. Amen!

I confess to you Jesus that I treated others like shit. I felt comfort when others suffered with me. Lord God, I give this up with your grace and help through faith in you Jesus.

This is connected to my pride: "that always keeps track of the score with me being on top. My well-being comes first so screw others. They don't matter". Lord God, I confess this as all wrong. Please forgive me. I give it up with your help through faith in you. Amen. [Done]

Lord God, this was all motivated by my fear that I will be the only one without the goodies. Lord God, I give this up with your help in faith confessing it to be horribly wrong. [You are forgiven Rene] Thanks Jesus!

Lord, this springs from my belief that life is unfair. I give this belief up with your help Jesus.

Lord God, I feel soft inside of me. Like I'm firing on all pistons of love. I care all of a sudden in my heart; not just in my mind anymore.

A little later the Lord made me aware of the following: I made the following commitment a long time ago: "I'm going to love myself and so is everyone else whether they like it or not." That became buried in my subconscious. This attitude often translated into me becoming selfish and putting myself first as well as meanly and abrasively demanding cooperation from others. Confessing this to God and repenting from it in prayer was key to helping me reclaim and recover more healthy love for people and pets.

8.3: The Great Pitfall Of Self-Pity

When a parent asks me to do a chore, or when a spouse asks me to do something (that Satan suggests with a lie is unfair), I can indulge in self-pity very easily. If I give into self-pity, then I am letting Satan spoil or steal a good deed that could have otherwise communicated to the parent or spouse that I love them. I'm determined to not let the devil steal my sense of positive purpose, healthy attitude, and helpful actions with self-pity. By indulging in self-pity in this context I would be treating the parent, spouse, and God as nuisances because of my compulsive-laziness and selfishness. When this dynamic is at work then I am treating people as task masters, or worse, as slave drivers who I am trying to appease with a certain quota of works so they will be happy (and get off my case) so I can go back to my own lazy ways. I need to repent in prayer from the self-pity, and counter the lies of the devil with liberating truth that will help me to love and go the extra mile instead.

Again, the battle against compulsive-laziness repeatedly needs to be tackled. But it does not have to remain a stronghold forever. We were wired for work, and work was prepared for us. Confession and repenting in prayer ought to be practiced repeatedly. And implementing the Golden Rule, in the context of grace, replaces the negative attitude of compulsive-laziness.

Not having a work ethic is one problem, but we can also go about being industrious the wrong way. This manifests in putting pressure on ourselves, hatred, anger, hostility, self-revenge or self-blackmail, malice, hitting oneself over the head, trying to conform to rules and commands (the minimum required quotas), angrily, tooth and nail, mercilessly, heartlessly, fearfully, hoping to earn favor from God by our efforts, hoping to find peace through our efforts, hoping to find freedom in our strengths, hoping to "find all the things" through doing "work" self-righteously through angry pressure instead of approaching work through a gentle faith in Jesus who offers grace freely.

This is often aided by an OT law mentality of "I must because the law says I must; otherwise I'm not a good person and am on my way to hell." The motivation becomes our fear. Writing these last two paragraphs has been difficult, because I have personally carried all these words and unhealthy motivations with me in one form or another. My heart and mind have been sick this way for way too long. Gently confessing it all along with its history, and repenting of it in prayer is the way forward. And it is conquered, not overnight, but in learning day in and day out about being in relationship with Jesus and seeking to do His will. We weren't given God's empowering presence to coldly obey a minimum standard. We are given the warm person of Jesus and His Spirit who comes alongside of us: to help us, to counsel us, and to urge us on to victory one battle at a time. Amen, and amen.

Focusing on a negative and passive set of laws—no matter how good—that try to bring fairness to protect our lower rights, will not motivate us to give to others or sacrificially love them, because then we are only looking for fairness for ourselves. But focusing on Jesus and gently submitting to His command to "go the extra mile" is fundamental to developing loving action. Action motivated by caring for people with our guilt washed away through confession and the power of bad habits broken through repentance and renewing the mind. Jesus does not invite us harshly, meanly, and angrily to go the extra mile. Jesus does not force us, or put pressure on us to keep His commands. He is kind and gentle. We need to speak to ourselves the way Jesus speaks to us. It is God's kindness that leads us to repentance.[35] We need to focus on Jesus and what He is saying to us. We cannot take the lonely road of an inner monologue with ourselves that achieves nothing but a stagnant, lifeless interior and a dead exterior relational life.

We need to start with being connected to what we care about and we find this place through two-way prayer to God. We can't care about everything. We all have different interests. We all have different gifts. We all have different opportunities. We all have different callings. We can't be all things to all people all the time. That is not realistic. But we can do something passionately useful, and with a caring heart: something greater than ourselves; something that has value in our eyes; something that calls us out of ourselves; something that helps other people feel good, full, relieved, at peace, hopeful, or like somebody cares; and something that makes us feel happy.

Compulsive-laziness or living in the "flesh" can be a mindset or a huge stronghold in one's life. Healthy people like accomplishing tasks at work, and with time off. Unhealthy people have no real goals in this life, and find false peace in doing absolutely nothing except possibly the bare minimum at work and home. Confessing and repenting from the "sin-conduit"-structures that contain laziness and/ or selfishness is a must if we want our love for others to grow and thrive.

8.4: Diagnosing And Healing Compulsive-Indulging

Compulsive-indulging also grows out of abandoning love in "the tree of knowledge of good and evil" within. When I am not willing to be active in love I will resent action unless it makes me feel good within a short enough time frame; the quicker the action the more likely it is to gratify me. Food and drink are quick and easy ways to feel good. The good I am *really* seeking is lasting peace. So if I only want to feel good, then compulsive-indulging will be a natural place to look in seeking peace independently from God.

The pathway to self-control is relationship with God. That means getting my bearings in conversation with God. Then in two-way prayer to construct Sin-Anatomy Tables for relevant Sin-Conduit Structures that wield power over my life. And, when the Holy Spirit gives consent, I then talk to God about the issues, sins, connections, and behaviors inserted in the Sin-Anatomy Tables as per the strategies (found in chapters 3 and 4) from this book. The repenting I do has to do with renewing my mind and giving up the lies I believe about what I am addicted to— whether it is food, drink, products, etc. This process deals with my past and guilt. And it gives me a new hope, a new start with a positive attitude, and a new strategy to live a healthier life.

Getting in touch with my feelings, attitudes, expectations, and energy behind my behaviors shows me what I am believing and thinking. This gives me a chance to see my fallen values.

---

[35] Cf. Romans 2:4

Putting to death the unhealthy believing and thinking and replacing it with positive submission to the teachings and commands of Jesus, this is key to victory—because Jesus' truth and grace sets us free. Nature hates a vacuum, so we have to replace the old bad habits with newer healthier habits. Anger is what I have improperly used in the past to motivate my change of habits. Recognizing this, confessing it to God, repenting from it, and then slowly steering my thoughts in healthier directions through prayer will help to complete the transformation. All negative emotions draw us towards finding relief rather than resolution transformation, and so beliefs that create negativity need to be put aside and replaced with healthy, warm, and happy ones.

To further replace the stronghold of compulsive-indulging with something healthier I need self-control—which is a fruit of the Holy Spirit. That means that it is a gift from the Holy Spirit. It is not a result of self-effort or self-will.

To help to protect against compulsive-indulging one needs to live within some healthy boundaries set up by God so that we stay away from unnecessary confusion that leads to temptations. Pursuing stillness and connection with God is the healthiest place to dwell through expectant faith as that is where the peace is. When you feel like compulsively eating then journal instead, because you are really hungry for God. [36] If your days go well by simply journaling in the morning, then think how healthy you will be when you follow through on journaling as a replacement for overeating. This helps us to commit to healthy thinking and values when it comes to what we eat and drink, and living for a purpose greater than pleasure like giving and receiving grace. Gluttony also has the effect of making us hate the perceptions we have of our bodies. This also needs to be confessed with the same intensity as it is felt. Gluttony is also hard on the pocketbook. Practically, wining this battle against compulsive-indulging daily will help us live within our budgets. If we only find short term freedom from compulsive-indulging through the steps outlined here, then we need to go deeper in prayer, build on truths we already know but have not utilized, and pray for new revelations. God does not give us a serpent when we ask for bread.[37]

Example: Tackling Compulsive-indulging

As a child I grew up enjoying food. But in my teens I remember buying plenty of junk food to gluttonize late at night to push away the boredom and emptiness I felt. In my university days, I became addicted to Coca-Cola but gave that up when I met Jesus. I remember one time hearing my friend voicing his concern about his belly and me laughing at him. But when I ended up being diagnosed with schizophrenia and being put on medication, I decided to use food to feel good as

---

[36] On how to journal I recommend Mark Virkler's books on journaling prayer.
[37] Cf. Mathew 7:9

little else did (this needed to be confessed to God and repented from too, and it did help to bring more self-control. Later, I had to go deeper by asking myself why I was so threatened emotionally when I thought about the possibility of my snacks being taken away from me (this led to working the coveting side of the Tree Diagram in this context and this brought more freedom from my food addictions)). I put on a lot of weight and so I then began to hate my body. This Sin-Conduit Structure has the form below along with its corresponding Sin-Anatomy Table beneath it:

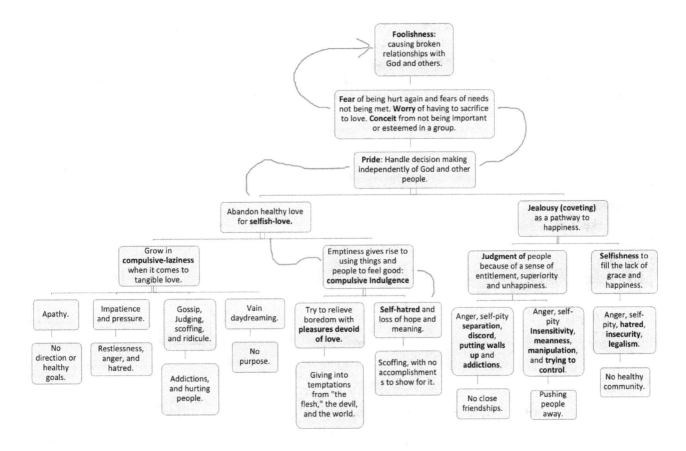

Frustration	Self-hatred	Over Eating	Abandoning Love	Pride	Fear	Foolish Judgment, & Sin
	<=	<=	<=	<=	<=	<= Cause and Effect
Tried to get happy with all sorts of gimmicks. Slave to food. Addiction demands more and more food with no return.	Disliked and hated my body. Am mean on myself using angry pressure as a means to stop eating junk food and drinking soda pop.	Set my heart on the pleasure of junk food to bring me happiness instead of loving people as myself.	Committed to pleasure seeking for decades with no consideration for what is healthy. Ignored God.	I see myself as the center of the universe. I know best by myself (don't need anyone else) on how to live my life.	Afraid of emptiness. How am I to fill the void inside?	As a teenager laughed at a friend's struggle with weight gain. Believed that pleasure is more important than truth and health.
I treated myself like this for decades						
Confession & Repenting in Faith =>	=>	=>	=>	=>	=>	

Prayer

"Lord Jesus, I confess my sin of hating my body and my insensitive judgment on my friend so long ago. I give up, through faith in you, my hatred of my body and judging people for their bodies. I receive your forgiveness and healing intellectually as well as emotionally. I confess my overeating as unhealthy, and I ask you to forgive me. I give this up along with attempting to use anger and self-pity to stop eating, with your help in faith, Jesus.

I admit pleasure seeking has been my goal for decades and not caring whether things are healthy or not; this is selfish-love that assumes pleasure is more important than health. I give up, with your help Lord Jesus, the lie that pleasure is more important than truth. It isn't. I'm sorry for living life on my own terms out of pride by trying to save myself or let food save me. I admit I'm afraid of emptiness and have believed the lie that I could fill it with whatever I wanted without consequences to my health and spirit.

Thank you for forgiving me and healing me. I invite you into my life into my emptiness, Jesus. I welcome you into that space of emptiness in my life Jesus with your peace and grace which surpasses all understanding. I choose to submit to you, and resist the devil. Please help me to think about what is healthy from now on, not be focused on selfish-love or try to motivate healthy actions through my anger or self-pity. Thank you, Jesus. Amen."

Dismantling Eating Unhealthily

I have a long, daily history of rushing myself in eating my food and trying to find the pleasure in it—wanting so much to feel consolation, pleasure and peace. The following is a diagnosis of where my eating habits have brought me:

1. **The Lie:** the faster I eat the more peace I feel.
2. **The repetition:** filling the emptiness over and over with the idols of food and drink.
3. **The hunger:** for peace, for meaning, and for happiness that is so elusive, because my strategy does not work. But I keep going back to it.
4. **The peace:** this is what I want most, and I am still seeking it in this area.

Prayer

"Lord God, I admit that I have forsaken you—the fount of life—for food and drink (pop, milkshakes, etc.) that are meant to give energy. But I used them as my substitute for you Lord God. Please forgive me. I'm sorry. I need you more than I know. I need you now. I needed you then. But I took what seemed most natural: milkshakes, burgers, fries, mayo, salt, buns, and ice cream to give me relief for short periods of time. Please forgive me for inhaling my food. I give it up now in faith, with your help and grace Lord Jesus. And I ask you the Holy Trinity to fill me instead with peace and life. For you are the beauty, majesty, peace, hope, and the desire of my life. I don't need to or want to inhale my food any longer. I choose to treat food with the respect it deserves. With your help Jesus, I ask for the gift of self-control to replace my compulsive-indulging. Thank you for your peace that is beyond description—that is what I really want, and I exchange my compulsive-indulging with your constant, caring presence, peace, and grace so I don't have to worship at the altar of food anymore. Amen."

More Healing of Compulsive-indulging

"Lord God, I confess that I have compulsive-indulging in my life in the form of eating unhealthily—not caring about the consequences and filling the void with pleasures that don't satisfy. Please forgive me and heal me of my sin. I give it up with your help through faith. I admit this comes from the selfish-love in my life and the willingness to use almost anything good or bad to bring consolation. I'm sorry and regret doing this. Please forgive me and heal this part of me with your touch. Thank you.

Lord I admit I do all of this out of pride which has these forms of thinking: "I know best," "I am most important in life," and "I am the center of the universe." I confess believing these lies, and I give them up with your help God through faith in you. I replace them with the truth that you are the center of the universe—not me. I'm sorry for looking down on others and ignoring your care and wisdom, Jesus. I ask for forgiveness and healing by trusting in your goodness and care, Father God. Thank you.

I am also motivated by fear. Fear of not finding or missing out on peace, consolation, entertainment, and excitement. Lord God, I give up these fears in faith, with your help now. I know that you care for everything you have created, and provide for our needs and many wants. Thank you for healing me.

I admit this compulsive-indulging started with foolishly turning away from you, the Fount of Life and the Living God. I ask your forgiveness for thinking I know better than anyone else on how to live life (mine and others). I'm sorry for rejecting you God and for my arrogance. I ask you into my life again. Please come into my void. I'm sorry for making such foolish decisions and living out this mentality for decades. Thank you for healing and forgiving me, Holy God. I am grateful you are in my life filling me with life, restoration, and peace. Amen."

Going Deeper

I had to do a lot of processing for my food and drink addictions. Here I went deeper still:

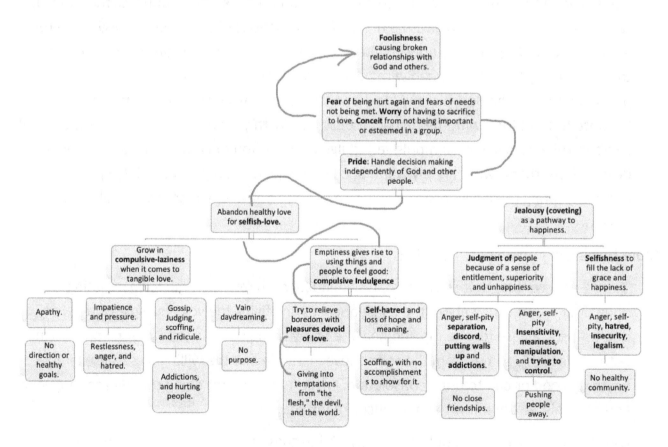

The above Sin-Conduit Structure has the following Sin-Anatomy Table:

Giving into fleshly temptation repeatedly	Compulsive Indulging	Abandoned Love	Pride	Fear	Foolishness
	<=	<=	<=	<=	<= Cause and Effect
Tried to relieve my pain, boredom and emptiness with food and drink.	Willing to use food and drink instead of approaching God for healing, love and life.	Ignored fellowship with God and sought to use food and drink to fill the void within.	I got to fill the void within at all costs while ignoring God and His wisdom.	Afraid my in most needs won't be met.	Separated myself from God's rich fellowship.
Did this for years without realizing the need to repent.					
Confession & Repenting in Faith =>	=>	=>	=>	=>	

Praying

Lord Jesus, I confess that I try to relieve my inner pain, boredom and emptiness with food and drink. This is idol worship. Please forgive me Lord Jesus. [Done] Lord Jesus I give up doing this with your help through your grace and through faith in you. [Done Rene]

Lord God, I admit that I seek to use food and drink to fill the void instead of approaching you for healing, love and life. I'm sorry! [Forgiven] Lord God, I come to you the Healer, Lover and Life giver of my whole existence refusing to ignore your place in my life any longer. I do so through your grace, Lord Jesus.

Lord God, I confess that I have abandoned fellowship with you and have sought to listen to the devil's lies about where I can fill my spiritual stomach. Please forgive me for doing this Lord God. [Done Rene] Lord God with your grace, truth and presence I choose to reject the devil's lies and empty promises. I choose with your help to fill my stomach with your life—your very self instead of the idols of food and drink.

Lord Jesus, I confess my pride that says I can fill my void and need to fill my void without letting you Lord God into the picture. Please forgive me Jesus. [Done] Lord Jesus, I give up my pride and choose to become teachable instead under you. Please help me to renew my mind/ heart/

thinking/ motives/ goals/ and focus with your grace through faith in you. [Done Rene]

Lord God, I confess that I have listened to the devil and so fears have filled my heart/ mind/ thoughts/ and attitudes; I'm afraid my in most needs won't be satisfied unless I seek to do it independently of you the Living God. Please forgive me for falling for this lie. [Done] Lord God I give up this fear with your help through faith and grace in you Jesus. Amen! [Answered]

Lord God I'm sorry for avoiding and ignoring you all these years in this area of my life. I renew my commitment to seek you, talk with you, listen to you and worship you alone as you deserve with your grace, truth and presence. Thank you, Lord God! Amen!

Going Deeper

Lord God, something that a drug addict said about his addiction stuck with me because I can relate to what he said despite the fact that I'm addicted to the feelings that food/ drink give me, not heroin. Lord, he said he loved how the drug made him feel. Nothing else gave him that feeling and he was willing to do whatever is needed to keep that feeling coming his way.

But why did I become a slave to food/ drink? The food/ drink offers me something I don't get anywhere else: special feelings. Lord, is this attraction, a root, part of a trunk, or a branch belonging to "the Tree of Knowledge of Good and Evil Within me"? [A root Rene!] So how do I give it up Jesus? [By confessing to Me, repenting in prayer, and breaking the attachment to the idols with words Rene]. Then let's do it Jesus!

Lord God, I confess I love how food/ drink make me feel. I have and do love it more than anything else including you oh God in this context. Lord God, please forgive me this sin. [Done!] I give up with your help and faith in you Jesus my commitment/ searching/ and grasping for the food/ drink that has given me the feelings I so prized. Thanks and Amen!

Lord Jesus, I break my addiction/ commitment to the feelings that comes from my food/ drink, with your grace, truth and presence. I have seen food and drink as the "cure-all" and "go-to" for decades starting at the beginning of my Dark Night. I have trusted its pleasure and the lie behind the pleasure: I can solve my problems by eating and drinking. I have wrongly valued it above all else in this context including you my God. I transfer my trust: that food/ drink (and the feelings I get from them) can solve my problems, to you Jesus. I have seen my food/ drink give me short term relief but cause more problems than it's worth. What a dead end. Lord God, I give up this commitment I made early in my Dark Night to attempt solving my problems with food/ drink with your help through faith in you Jesus. Amen and Amen.

8.5: Stability, Self-Control, And Resources

Seeking to do God's will is so important to stabilizing us. If the above strategy does not dislodge the stronghold of compulsive-indulging, then looking at my book *Going Deeper With The Twelve Steps,* which includes two chapters on Cycles of addiction, can be very helpful. If these don't help then going deeper in prayer (because God is deeper still) is the path to take.

Self-control comes from being at rest inside of us; this comes from the peace the Holy Spirit gives. The Holy Spirit's gift of self-control also comes as we learn to think and believe more healthily and trust Jesus to save us from our sins. We are enabled to love and value people, nature and healthy tasks instead of finding unhealthy, empty happiness in creature comforts. In submitting to God, we seek His will which is higher than ours, and that means seeking to think and act healthily in our decisions. This is called walking in holiness.

Sometimes, confessing the struggle to God and simply speaking directly to the "sin nature" when compulsive-indulging is at the door will suffice: saying, "I accept you, but I don't need you right now"; praying, "I give it up with your help Jesus through faith"; and inviting Jesus' grace and peace into our empty space to set us free to love and not sin. These prayerful steps give us self-discipline and self-control to conquer the temptation. As for food, eating healthily instead of eating to lose weight is wiser.

After the spiritual medicine has been applied and healing has come, then the next step is to give up the belief (in spite of years of powerlessness) that we still can't practice self-control and self-discipline. We must start believing we can again with the Holy Spirit's help. We must get up and start to practice self-discipline together with self-control with the ability God is gradually giving us as new life and hope flows into our lives.

Praying the prayers in this book might help a lot initially, but as we forget and gradually squeeze out Jesus' presence (along with His peace) wherever He can be found in our lives, then we will fill the void with idols instead (nature hates vacuums, and self-control will elude us). The Bible says Jesus has been crucified since the foundation of the world. I believe that this—in part— means that fallen humanity tries to mutilate the image of God that we are created in (within us), and substitute it with things that can't give life. The Bible says that Jesus is the way. I interpret this to mean that He is the way to love, peace, meaning, and purpose. We have to pursue Jesus daily in order to grow in loving God more fully and our neighbors as ourselves. This will help to humble our selfish-love along with its progenies: compulsive-laziness, and compulsive-indulging.

Learning to pursue Jesus takes a lifetime. Sometimes He hides from us so that we will feel our spiritual hunger and thirst more keenly, and this helps us to then pursue Him more passionately, truthfully, and gracefully.

In this book, I have not exhausted all the reasons for people not having self-control (sometimes observing certain healthy eating habits needs to be incorporated, as well as doing exercise that is not work related). Medications can also have side effects such as weight gain. If these medications are necessary to live a normal life then the weight gain needs to be watched and fought off as much as it is in our power to do so. When we have done everything we know to quit (i.e. searched more deeply in prayer), but just can't seem to get over that hump in our path, then we need to put our faith in Jesus to save us and wait (search even more deeply) for His truth and grace to set us free. Jesus is a reliable Savior; He will never leave us nor forsake us even when life seems absurd.

9 Diagnosing & Healing My Coveting Branches Of The Tree Of Knowledge Of Good And Evil Within

Coveting grows out of pride on the right side of "the tree of knowledge of good and evil". Many times we can covet good things but use unhealthy means to attain them—which is what the "tree of knowledge of good and evil" gets us to do. Coveting means we care more about our concerns than the people in the way. Coveting also has the meaning of seeking things that others don't necessarily have, but that we want and think we deserve: our feather in the hat, our jewel in our crown, and what amounts to our elevated status in the community.

Coveting can be jealous and envious. Envy sees God as a miser. It is blind to grace, devoid of grace, and so wrongly blames God for the supposed lack in our lives. Envy is negative in nature and by itself can force a person to seek relief through other means and therefore also starts addictions like eating comfort food. Envy is a jealous and hateful attitude. It demands being first when it comes to the loyalty others show, or to have the best attributes or abilities when compared to others. Jealousy is more about getting things we want than getting a better reputation. When we have envy and jealousy they are both aimed at people who have something we don't have. Self-pity can be envy and jealousy's servant.

Repeated, pointed, accurate, gentle, and genuine prayer is central to help breaking these strongholds through grace. If we are envious of a person, then like Pope Francis advises: give thanks to God in prayer for being so generous with the gifts He gave to the persons we envy. This works if we respect God, are receiving His grace, and are open to sharing it. Faith in a good and generous God also helps to kill the stronghold of envy in us. Also, giving thanks to God helps kill envy and *actually* aids us in being generous.

We begin by finding our bearings, and start a two-way dialogue with God in an attempt to construct Sin-Anatomy Tables for relevant Sin-Conduit Structures. In the "broken relationships and foolishness" column we deal with our histories (conflicts, attacks, and unhealthy loyalties and beliefs). And then proceed to fill out the rest of Sin-Anatomy Table for the relevant Sin-Conduit Structure. We dismiss through prayer jealousy and envy's servants: self-pity, anger, and pressure in the right contexts for freedom to come.

Then we process the Sin-Anatomy Tables as per the strategies (from chapters 3 and 4) in this book.

Being open to the Holy Spirit as we learn to think more healthily and trust Jesus to save us from our jealousy. He enables us to love as we put aside jealousy by saying yes to grace and thanksgiving. But we need to be mindful of where we are at, fight with truth, and not try to wrestle our self-pitying feelings all by ourselves with carnal forceful energy. Instead we fight with strategic prayer, gentle wisdom, genuine prayer and faith in Jesus that brings grace and unconditional love into our lives. These allow us to help care for others and deny jealousy when it tries to reassert itself, so that my mind and attitudes are slowly renewed with little "t" truths and grace.

Jesus calls us to altruism—to seeking the highest good of those we meet. Jesus calls us to love others like ourselves. When we are purely absorbed with only our own whims, cares, and personal desires, always watching that things are fair, with self-pity when we don't get our own way—we are not happy campers, and live in the "flesh" not the Spirit. The "flesh" and the Spirit are opposed: the flesh can't please the Spirit and the "flesh" can't submit to the Spirit.

We are designed to give unselfishly and so feel happiest when we do so and share in the mind of Christ. We find meaning and purpose in giving honor, respect, and value to others; but happiness is fleeting when we are hoarding position and power for ourselves. Position and wealth won't fill the void within.

Moving towards seeing people as treasures, as opposed to earthly wealth and position, is a journey worth taking. People who get this are usually the happiest of us all; they value, receive, and give grace. We get there by understanding grace and welcoming it into our lives daily through communion with God through Jesus Christ.

Sometimes when some of the roots have been uprooted in a certain Sin-Conduit Structure we can still go to an ugly place when certain challenges come our way. It is sort of like a chicken running about with its head cut off doing its own thing; and in such cases an "Event + Reaction = Outcome" strategy may be needed.

The time between an event and its outcome is the place where we decide what we want and how we ought to react. This is important, because it says we do have time and don't have to always make quick decisions. Quick decisions are not always wise; they can be made in foolishness, blindness, fear and panic, and so bring the same old, unwanted results.

When our wills are still engaged in old reactive behaviors (by default or leftover deception) despite the fact that the compulsive energy is now gone through dismantling, then we must ask ourselves when we are challenged, "Do I still want to go to this old place?" And if not, then we are free to change our reactions slowly with new thinking—redirecting our wills, and therefore avoiding the old bad habits—thereby making our repentance more complete. For example, if we are mean when we are angry. We can then jettison the meanness and process the anger without sinning.

9.2: Diagnosing And Healing Judging And Unhealthily Motivated Anger

Judging grows out of pride in "the tree of knowledge of good and evil." When somebody does something that we dislike, then in judging them, we may do any of the following: accuse, insinuate, label, call them names, castigate, use hateful and negative speech, cast a bad light on them, hurt them, or make them angry. This may make them want to defend themselves, and judge us back out of anger. But when we tell the truth, we will use "I" statements.

In repenting from judgments we need to expose the lies behind the judgments we make and replace them with truth in order to become free. For instance, if we believe and endorse that people deserve being laughed at when they do something stupid, then we will laugh at them whenever they do something stupid in our eyes. Just praying, "I say no to my judging of 'so and so' with your help Jesus" does not go far enough. We must get specific—get to the roots, and expose the unhealthy commitments, values, and lies we are holding onto behind the judgments. We must confess them to God and repent from them in prayer in order for freedom to result.

We can say something like, "I don't like this person," and think there is nothing wrong with doing so, but it can have a range of (acceptable to unacceptable) meanings or energies beneath it: we're unhappy about what the person did; we dislike the person's attitude; we don't approve of the person; we're angry with this person; we don't want to be around the person; we choose to harden our hearts towards the person; we're against the person; we hate what the person did; we hate the person; we want the person to hurt; we want the person banished; we want the person killed; (or worse) I'm going to kill the person. These unacceptable judgments need to be repented from in order to be free of the bad energy.

Having malice in our hearts can be hard to detect and written up as just an anger problem. But I have found that judging and anger can be triggered by a general commitment in my affairs to repaying evil for evil. Giving up this revenge mentality with Jesus' help in faith *really* helps us respond to disappointments, broken expectations, and potential boundary violations, with kindness, tolerance, and forgiving attitudes and behaviors.

I now know that healthy anger is like an signal. When we have it, it says something is wrong within or outside of me that needs to be addressed. I may feel injustices of rights being violated, may think my expectations are not being met, or I may believe my supposed entitlements have been compromised when I feel anger. What I believe may need to be reassessed and repented from when what I believe does not reflect reality, truth or honesty, or does not foster healthy relating.

I have learned that if I believe my anger is immoral, then I will get angry with myself for my anger, and that just screws me up interiorly to the point of confusion, self-pity, exasperation and more anger. These blind me to what the real issues really are.

When judging causes or increases my anger, then dealing with the judging will clear up much of the anger. Judgment ought to be a short-term visitor not a long-term house guest (i.e. it shouldn't become a resentment). Anger that is not relieved or dealt with in healthy ways will poison my mind, heart, speech, and energy. It compromises my connectedness because I'm likely using it to try to get my own way. Also, anger that is not dealt with and is hidden away turns into resentments, addictions, hostility, bitterness, insensitivity, and hatred. It needs to be addressed if we want to be healthy spiritually.

Given that we are allowed to be angry with others when injustices occur, it follows that others are allowed to be angry with me too. Anger is about how one feels when one perceives an injustice. We need to set people free to process their anger. And we ought to process our anger healthily too. We can't necessarily go around telling people they ought not be angry. And we shouldn't stuff or bury our own anger either.

Injustices happen, happen often, and cause anger. There are those injustices that happen because people are led that way by the devil and then there are those things that are systemic— inherent to the created order, marred by sin and having pushed God away, causing frustration, headaches, confusion, pain, anger and torment. There is no sense in blaming God because our darkness can't cast out darkness.

9.3: A Healthy Way To Deal With Anger And Broken Expectations

When I have expectations that aren't being met, then the unhealthy thing to do is to get stuck (i.e. become full of self-pity, pout, or use the tool of anger on the person who has triggered me because I want something from the person). Sometimes my anger is so hidden because my self-pity is so strong emotionally. If I feel self-pity then often anger and pressure are there too—and vice-versa; meaning both need to be addressed in prayer.

The healthy thing to do when we're told no by somebody when we are expecting a yes is to respect the person and give up the sought after expectation (with Jesus help through faith in prayer). If it is blocking our love for the person, then we need to accept that the person in question has said no, and then move onto loving those people in the situation that triggered the anger. Recalibrating our expectations regularly sets others and ourselves free from dogmatism and so it is very healthy for all the people involved.

When I have expectations that are not met, instead of just getting angry, I can also judge the person who did not come through for me. And the inclination is to think I need to forgive the person who did not meet my expectations. But what I *really* need to do is repent in prayer from my judging so that I can find peace. Judging people is always wrong. I'm learning that using "I" statements in telling the truth can be helpful in processing my worries in non-judgmental ways, and it helps to set me free from confusion and burdens.

Most people do their best in what they seek to achieve. Acknowledging this is one way to not get nitpicky, anal, negative, and judgmental.

9.4: Dealing With Anger And Rejection

In dealing with anger, rejection is a *big deal*. In speaking about Jesus, an OT writer said, "He was rejected and despised by people... familiar with pain..."[38] When I am rejected I can handle it in my own fallen way or in Jesus' way. My ways have been many: to not process it at all; to try to push it down; to get and stay angry (when I was very young); to plot getting even through withdrawal; and to pretend nothing happened at all because I felt such deep pain (note: when I pretend, then I am putting on a mask, and I do so because I think it will save me from my shame and make me look strong). None of these feel good or are healthy, and steal from our true vocation as humans. And it often can get laminated onto how we view reality in a really unhealthy way. I now know how to process rejection, anger, and pain in a healthy way thanks to Jesus. This means not being a masochist and not being a doormat either.

When I inflexibly demand my rights without giving people choice, then I am asking for rejection, defiance, and on my part low self-esteem and getting stuck emotionally from a lot of no's from all the people I will disagree with. When I go this route, I use dark, negative energy, and things get ugly. Giving people a way out through dialogue to express where they are at and to what they can commit to (or not) is a more humble and flexible path to take.

The person who can't take a no for an answer may be stubbornly selfish, envious, conceited and proud. If this is the case, then they have problems accepting that others have a right to say no. Because of this they are prone to ugly, angry outbursts and plenty of self-pity. This needs to be healed through the medicines found in Jesus: His presence, grace, and truth.

Jesus was rejected to the point of being crucified and left for dead. Jesus handled rejection not by going to a place of resentment but by pouring Himself out in love from death to resurrection: treating us with care (He said, "They know not what they do"), and forgiving us (He said, "Father forgive them"), and declaring, "It is finished," when it came to our forgiveness. Jesus did not run from His pain, hide from His accusers, say He deserved it, or numb His pain. He navigated the pain by caring for people, by loving people, and focusing on the joy set before Him. Jesus did not see the cross as a problem but an opportunity to show His love to the full. Rejection is not the end of life as we know it. There is life after rejection, and when we navigate rejection healthily, there is joy waiting for us. The anger does not have to be eternal.

I have found that when I had the fear of rejection (with walls coming up when triggered) it was rooted in hurts and rejection in my past. Tracing the paths in "the tree of knowledge of good and evil," that maps out this fallen structure within me, we can then pray through them all the way to the roots (possible instigated or reactionary sin (on my part), the hurts inflicted, and fears). Confessing and repenting in prayer of my personal sins (including bad commitments and

---

[38] Isaiah 53:3

misguided loyalties), forgiving the agents of my hurts, along with replacing lies with truth is the healthy path to take. We then go deeper in prayer if the fear of rejection gets triggered again. The root might have many branches. For me, I realized later that I aimed for perfection thinking if I'm perfect then no one will reject me. No one is perfect; and God gets rejected even though He is perfect. I had to confess this dynamic to God and give it up with Jesus' help in prayer. When this is dealt with other triggers can be dealt with too if they exist.

I have found that raised walls in me, after I've been rejected, get lowered when I deal healthily with the remnants of conceit that get triggered. When I do struggle with rejection, praying through conceit and fear as outlined in this book, and renewing my mind with the truth that God loves me, does help me to move on in positivity and kindness. Walls then come down so that I'm able to care for the people in my life.

9.5: Anger And Complete Compliance

Anger often comes from a "religious" person because they perceive that the law has been broken in some context, that people are on their way to hell because of it, and that voicing anger for the sin will somehow bring repentance. I have struggled with this mentality personally for a long time.

I now have a better grasp on it thanks to this revelation that broke into my mind: the law expects complete compliance; I'm not the law, so I shouldn't expect it from others or myself, because when I expect it I'm always angry, inflexible, hard, unkind, rigid, ungracious, and unhappy. This brought some freedom and breathing room in my life, but it slowly eroded as I felt we still needed some sort of standard to live by instead of what looked more and more like a license to sin. But then I asked myself, "Am I under law or grace?" The answer was obvious: "I'm under grace." So, if I'm not under the law, then how can I expect perfect compliance to the law from others? Is there now no standard at all for anyone?

I believe there are standards. For me, the standards are Jesus' commands found in the NT which are much higher than the OT Law. And in living out Jesus' commands the law is *actually* fulfilled through His grace. So no matter what people do, according to Jesus' standard, I'm asked to love people unconditionally. This is what Jesus asks me to do. And it does away with the expectation within me of perfectionism from others and myself. Grace is deciding to love somebody whether or not they do good, do bad, or are indifferent. I like it when people are that way to me, so I want to be that way to them: "Do to others what you want them to do to you," which is the Golden Rule. Mental assent to this rule is not good enough; we have to choose to live it out with Jesus' grace when the opportunity makes itself present.

We live out grace by dealing with sinful strongholds or triggers (usually my past sins, foolishness, judgments, unhealthy loyalties and beliefs). The gateways to healing these triggers are to process my visible sins that are connected via Sin-Conduit Structures and process these as outlined and suggested (in chapters 3 and 4) in this book. Each stronghold has a theme, and we just have to ask the right questions to God and ourselves to fill in the 'in between' blanks.

As a temporary measure we can also say to the sin energy of anger and self-pity in the context of judging, "I accept you but I don't need you right now," and pray, "I give this up, with your help Jesus, through faith." Then we submit to God, resist the devil by processing the relevant Sin-Conduit Structures and seek to live out of Jesus' grace instead of judging.

But what about those not under God's grace? They have consciences just like anyone else. For some people, they embrace the law (which was God's minimum OT standard), and this helps them until they discover grace. Even those without the OT written Law are created in God's image and so they have some sense of right and wrong (often better than mine).

Jesus said that the Holy Spirit would convince the world of sin so it is not my responsibility or job to convict others of sin or be a moral policeman. Jesus said for me to not judge or condemn people. When I'm angry at someone it is because I have judged the person. When I've judged I have used a standard that I don't even keep perfectly myself so I am judged because I have, in pride, put myself above another—and so I'm also a hypocrite.

So grace and the Golden Rule set me free from judging and anger that come from the expectations of complete compliance tied to the law (and personal, anal codes of conduct).

Trying to put out a fire by trying to blow away the smoke is not smart; we can do this with anger a lot of the time trying to control it, stashing it away, or wrestling with it. But we should not feel guilty about the actual anger when it acts like a warning signal; we just need to process it healthily. In this context, anger is a sign that we need to act and be responsible for our jealousy and judging. Fear leads to pride. Pride leads to jealousy and jealousy to judging. Judging leads to anger or even rage. Rage can very easily birth hatred too. So getting rid of and processing my foolish loyalties, fear, pride, jealousy/ coveting, and judging will help get rid of and process my anger in this context.

When our boundaries are violated or people get into our personal spaces the "sin nature" can or will rear its ugly head and try to use anger and self-pity to resolve the violation. I have found that when we're put into such situations we can do the following: simply confess the struggle to God; speak directly to our "sin nature" saying, "I accept you, but don't need you right now"; pray "I give this up, with your help Jesus, through faith"; and invite Jesus' peace in to overcome the sin within, lift me above the dark pull, and enable me to love unconditionally. We are thereby equipped by the Holy Spirit to give grace instead of immature intolerance to the people who triggered us to feel uncomfortably mean and full of unkindness.

Practicing principles can sometimes become like trying to uphold the law and we end up feeling powerlessly adrift. I have learned that when principles don't seem to have any power, then I need a new start and need to put my faith in Jesus to save me because there are things I'm not seeing that Jesus does. And when I do put my faith in Him, He always comes through eventually.

9.6: Anger, Law, And Grace

Law focused people only get angry, and think God agrees with their indignation, when they see people individually or communally walking away from God into sin. And if only the angry belief remains in them (that the people deserve hell), then such people remain law focused. Jeremiah was an OT prophet called "the weeping prophet" because he connected with where God was emotionally as the Jewish people of his time lived out the consequences of their sins. When we weep over a person's separation from God, then we are grace focused and have the heart of Jesus. Jesus weeps tears of living water, also known as the Holy Spirit or Love.

In the parable of the prodigal son, the father (representing God) is not full of wrath when the younger son claims his inheritance and walks off into sin. Rather the father knows the boy is unwise, immature and doesn't know how good he has it. So the father—in love—gives the boy his inheritance and lets him go off to seek his fortune. The father knows that the lessons learned will bring him back to sanity when he remembers how good the father really was and is. And that story symbolizes what happens often between us and God.

9.7: Anger And Judgment That Inevitably Leads To Addictions

Pride and jealousy both spawn unhealthily motivated anger in "the tree of knowledge of good and evil" within. Pride and jealousy are very hard on others. If we have anger issues and don't forgive, then judging leads to resentments. The anger we feel towards the person will be justified in our eyes and will create negativity, emptiness, discord, sourness, coldness, hardness, depression, and bitterness. But since we were made for joy, we will seek to nurse these negative feelings with pleasures if we don't forgive, and this will create compulsions towards whatever pleasures come first. My book *Going Deeper With The Twelve Steps* is a constructive way to forgive and deal with such addictions.

When we forgive, the negative burden lifts, the anger is given up, and the judgment is lifted. But we are not free yet. If our jealousy, pride, conceit, and self-pity are not dealt with, then we will fall into judging repeatedly as well as into the addiction—and no one wants that. Therefore, we need to deal with the hurt or foolishness, the conceit and self-pity, the fear, the pride, and the jealousy (the Sin-Conduit Structure) in our hearts with the medicine mentioned above. When these are dealt with regularly we will find less time and money being spent on our addictions and more on others. Hence, giving will become a way of life. With freedom from addictions we will move onto the way of love—which is Jesus.

9.8: Anger And A Demanding Spirit

When we have a demanding spirit it means we are—whether hidden or revealed—harsh, angry, without good will, nasty, and forcefully expecting others to comply with our wishes as though it is an unquestionable, divine right. The energy is ugly, the attitude is jerk-like, and it does not respect the people it is aimed at.

I am convinced that we can't demand things from others what we think will make us happy. That includes everyone in our life. If we demand it then it is no longer a gift and isn't done in freedom, joy, hope, and altruism. So what about our expectations? What sort of place do they have? Do we have to watch ourselves carefully from crossing over from expecting to demanding? Yes, we do.

After trying to love from my heart and learning to practice humility in brokenness, pain and suffering for years, I went through a disorientating "woe is me" and "nothing satisfies" period. I was unable to *really* focus on meaningful goals: having no altruistic motivation, having a parched interior life, nurturing feelings of unfairness, feeling a desire to accuse God, and lacking the power to love—basically having no wind in my sails.

I felt depressed and sad—like all my efforts were futile. Knowing what I wanted I could not demand from others: God first, family second, and friends next. Because when I demand (which is negative in nature) I seek my own, which is not what love is. And if people comply, then there is a good chance it isn't done freely, genuinely, healthily, and caringly when they respond to my bad energy. I'd rather people be genuinely caring than doing things out of a guilt trip instigated by me, out of some sense of obligation, out of fear of my anger or my disapproval, or out of fear of me rejecting them for not complying with my wishes.

I found it freeing to pray through all the instances I was involved in where I had a demanding spirit. A person with a strong demanding spirit does not bend easily, pouts a lot when they don't get their way, and manages to find convenient excuses to not go the extra mile. I've been this person before many times.

How do demanding spirits gain their foothold in us? They start out with expectations, and their power is enhanced when fear, self-pity, anger, pride, and selfishness come into the picture through foolishness. It is self-preservation gone bad. Giving up these expectations along with my foolishness, fear, self-pity, anger, pride, and selfishness is fundamental to giving up a demanding spirit.

9.9: Anger And Judgment That Leads To Shallowness

God's love is not coercive. He does not threaten or use force to get people to choose Him or His ways. Our love is real when it is not motivated by the possibility of punishment, wrath, anger, and threats of hell. There are boundaries that God has set in place regarding acceptable moral behavior, and He warns us of the consequences of walking outside those limits. But God does not come down hard on us because we sin. Instead sin has its own inherent consequences, because we usually reap what we sow—except for grace and mercy. The idea that God is some kind of angry, cosmic, police enforcer needs to be set aside for another root of judgmental attitudes to be uprooted and to help peace reign in our hearts. Those who live under the threats of their god, live under fear and may very well be inclined to judge other people, because that is the way they experience life.

In having success against judgmental attitudes we need to be wary of, and let go of, seeing God as coercive. When we see God as Love, then it is easier to work through our anger or judgmental strongholds as described here.

When I have an unhealthily motivated anger (defined as being rooted in the Sin-Conduit Structure of: foolishness, resentment, or judgment leading to fear, self-pity and conceit, leading to pride, leading to jealousy, and leading to a judging mentality), I will forever be drawing lines in the sand unless the structure can be dismantled. By that I mean that I won't find pleasure in people too easily; I may very well hate them or be unable to love them because of blockages in my thinking and heart. I will have this negative energy fueling me and it will push me away from others and them from me. This will only validate my belief that people deserve my judgments, and I possibly end up being a hypocrite too because I let things slide when I do the same things that pisses me off when others do them. Hence, I will have less intimacy, be more insensitive, and tend to isolate from others. I will not be able to value people for who they are and that means I will have superficial relationships.

The truths I have found that help to silence judging are: sincerely believe that everyone is special in their own way, and to see the line between good and evil as going through each person's heart and not between empires, traditions, cultures, groups, and people; and to give up a "we are good vs. they are evil" mentality.

To get rid of my judgmental attitude, I must understand the difference between judging and telling the truth. "Giving an opinion about *someone else* is judging, whereas giving my honest opinion about *myself* is truth telling."[39] The reason why I am very tempted into thinking judgmental thoughts and to want to follow through on judging people is because I feel injustices have been visited on me. Even when I recognize that Jesus commanded me to not judge, I am pulled in a way to try to make things right, because I think that if I don't speak up things will get worse. This tension occurs because I don't know how to speak my truth gently. Judging attacks others, whereas speaking the truth does not. Truth speaking involves using "I" statements that own my feelings in conversations with those who hurt me; these statements are more likely to illicit understanding and change (although those who don't care may laugh me off). Whereas,

---

[39] Danny Silk, used with permission.

when I judge, then I blame and put people on the defensive—and this will not bring healing. Healing of the relationship will come only if there is forgiveness and understanding on both sides.

Years ago, I was promised an opportunity that was not coming through for me. I was tempted to get bitter and hostile, and I had many judgmental thoughts towards the person I thought was responsible for reneging on his promise. But when it came time to confront the person I did not blame him—I did not vent, hate, scream injustice, or judge the person—I just said how I felt. A few days later the opportunity came my way. I now know the person did not feel judged by me, and he was warmed by my response to his cold shoulder. I see this as a powerful example of the difference between judging and telling the truth.

Again, to cure our judgmental attitudes fully we will need to be healed from all the negative attitudes (conceit, self-pity, anger, judgments, fear, arrogance, pride and jealousy that are in our hearts) by using the medicines from this book. In curing these we will peel away the superficial exterior surrounding our lives and people will be attracted to our positive energy. To stay free and love supernaturally we need to care for people more, grow in thankfulness, and trust in Jesus.

After we have done a lot of work dismantling the strongholds of pride and related attitudes (such as judging), we will have more clarity and connectedness in our minds. We will be able to see just how immature our old thought-patterns, attitudes, and desires are after working through "the tree of knowledge of good and evil" diagram with strategic prayer as outlined in this book.

Certain situations will trigger certain thoughts, and those thoughts will trigger these immature, black-and-white, reactions and attitudes that threaten to explode in the present. These are reactions to instances that were not handled healthily or properly in the past. For the longest time, I still wanted to go to a place of childish judgment in certain areas, and I realized I needed to use "I" statements to healthily process my feelings in these areas. Sometimes that is all it takes, but sometimes I need to examine my negative beliefs and thoughts behind the judgment that triggered my immature meltdowns. I can then trade them in for wise, mature, and realistic beliefs and thoughts of gentleness, kindness, and patience—which leads to peaceful expressions of relating to the people and situations that were triggers in the first place. All this positivity is made possible through confession and repenting in faith with Jesus' help, teachings, commands, and promises. Grace and truth, along with the person of Jesus giving Himself to me continually, propels me ahead. It does not work if we only give mental assent to these truths. We have to trust it all, in the face of all the negative, mean, hostile, bitter, self-pitying attitudes and beliefs, and to choose to dispense grace to others instead.

There are certain things that parents and siblings do to us in childhood that can trigger immature reactions even now in our adulthood. Confessing our baggage and giving up these reactions in prayer (i.e. judging, whining, complaining, or being hostile, cold, and mean) will help us to get rid of our emotional baggage and set us free from being triggered into choosing immature behaviors.

9.10: Anger And Judgment That Leads To Moral Policing

Another bad fruit from jealousy is that I will become mean, territorial, and intolerant towards those who cross my boundaries and do things I find immoral. This is where learning about compassion and non-violence as a pathway to resolving disputes that Jesus championed is so very important. This can only be done through truth and grace. The meek are slow to anger, and knowing how to channel anger is so invaluable. But jealousy will produce intolerance, and this needs to be dealt with first (along with the pride, fear, and self-pity in our hearts as found in "tree of knowledge of good and evil" within). Humility is what will result, and it will help give me love for my enemy—that leads to healing broken relationships or resolving conflicts.

Moreover, taking a close look at the tone and energy in our speech is also important. Do we call people derogatory names (if not to their face perhaps behind their backs)? Is there meanness in our words? Is there self-pity behind our words? Do we put people down? Do we hurt people with our words? Do we rob hope from people? Are we hostile? Do we try to manipulate others to try and get our own way? Do we use judgmental words with others before listening and speaking to them? If so, then we have corrupt tongues.

For me, knowing that it is God's kindness that leads me to change for the better is helping me in how I treat others, because if it works for God, then it will work for my relationships too.

This is the path to take: confessing to God and owning the developmental history of these vices and bad fruits in my life, receiving forgiveness and healing in faith, repenting in prayer from this stronghold, and renewing one's mind with healthy truth and grace. We must submit to God and resist the devil. Changing how one speaks won't happen overnight, but it can be done gradually through heartfelt prayer, as truth and wisdom and grace come into play.

Understanding and embracing the grace that comes from God, and abandoning my attachments to my lower rights and dark impulses for personal justice to be meted out at every turn will all help to tame moral policing and make me open and strong in kindness. Love does not seek its own interests.

The NT calls us to believe the best about those we meet.[40] When we do this we see people as having been made in the image of God: that they were made for God, that they are called to

---

[40] Cf. 1 Corinthians 13:1-13

love, and that Jesus' intention towards them is altruistic, caring, and hope filled in nature. Nothing changes out of loading people down with guilt. Supernatural change comes from grace, kindness, caring, and seeing people the way God does—with love. If we act mean to a person who is mean in order to try to get them to change for the better, then we are deluded.

Saying yes to the Golden Rule, in the context of dispensing grace, and accepting God's will are powerful medicines meant to replace judgmental attitudes and actions with restorative justice and mercy.

Anger can show up in us when others withhold what we mistakenly think we justly deserve. Like when we do something wrong to someone, and we confess and apologize to the person, but they don't immediately forgive us. But we don't deserve to be forgiven. We need to allow others to process the hurts we inflict on them and to journey to forgiveness in their own time. Love is not coercive. Love sets people free with no manipulation, threats, or strings attached. Yes, Jesus requires them to forgive but that is between them and Him. Jesus has taught me that we shouldn't judge or condemn. The Holy Spirit will convince others, and we don't have to go around and preach condescendingly to them or try to win over people through guilt, anger, shame, and fear. Blessed are the merciful for they will receive mercy. God convinces us through His kindness, with neither anger nor hostility. We need to use our spiritual mirrors to see where we ourselves are at.

Example: Giving Up Judgment of "Me vs. Them"

The following is a Sin-Conduit Structure with the Sin-Anatomy Table written beneath it:

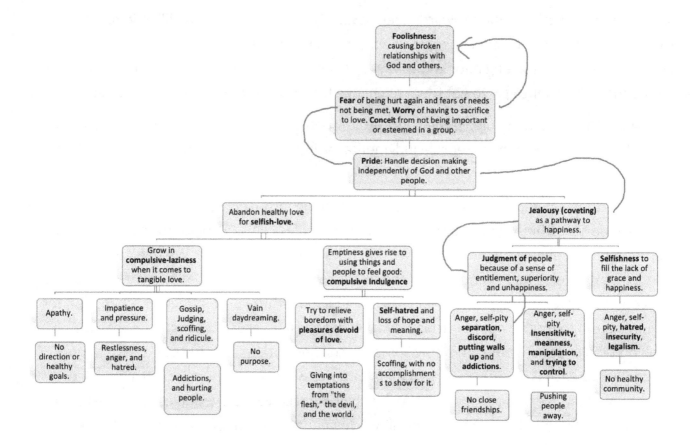

Loneliness	Judging	Covering & Envy	Pride & Rebellion	Fear & Conceit	Foolishness & Judging
	<=	<=	<=	<=	<= Cause and Effect
Isolation, no friends, cynical, jaded, critical, nice to nice people; mean to unfriendly people. Chip on shoulder.	"Me=smart vs. Them=stupid". I hate them, I'm better than them.	I want what they have: being in the in crowd. Why don't I belong like they do? I'll show them.	I'm better than them. No one will ever hurt me again. Lots of self-pity and angry pressure used on me by me to never let me hurt like what happened again.	Fear of me being hurt again. Have a poor me, and self-pity attitude.	Being hard on myself out of reactions to foolish failures, rejection, hurt. Blamed those who rejected me.
Confession & Repenting in Faith=>	=>	=>	=>	=>	

Praying Through It

"Lord Jesus, I confess my judgment, envy, pride, cowardly fear, hurt, foolishness, and deceitfulness in the context of all my relationships. With your help I give up the following: judging people by thinking "I'm smart" and "they're stupid"; my envy which says I want to belong at all costs; my pride that says: "I'm better than they think"—which wrongly insinuates they are judging me; my fear of being hurt again, because it isn't the end of the world being hurt by rejection when I handle it in a healthy way; and my self-pity, anger, and pressure that I direct squarely onto myself to be perfect. With your help Jesus, I forgive myself, and I receive your forgiveness and healing in this area of my life both intellectually and emotionally. Lord God, I ask that you replace my intolerance with kindness, warmth, and caring humility. Thank you for being here for me and being constantly non-judgmental. You inspire me to love people because you are beautiful to me. Amen."

As far as judging is concerned we can have a "me vs. them" mentality (that is reversed) where we take the short end of the stick instead of a place of *supposed* glory. We can have this negative mentality or box that we try to box out of because of other people's judgments against us that we might wrongly embrace as a part of our identities. This also needs to be prayed through by forgiving those who called us names (we may need to forgive ourselves too) in order for spiritual health to be restored in such an area.

Another example with the following sin conduit. In this situation I was driven to compulsively discount other people's feelings thinking I knew better.

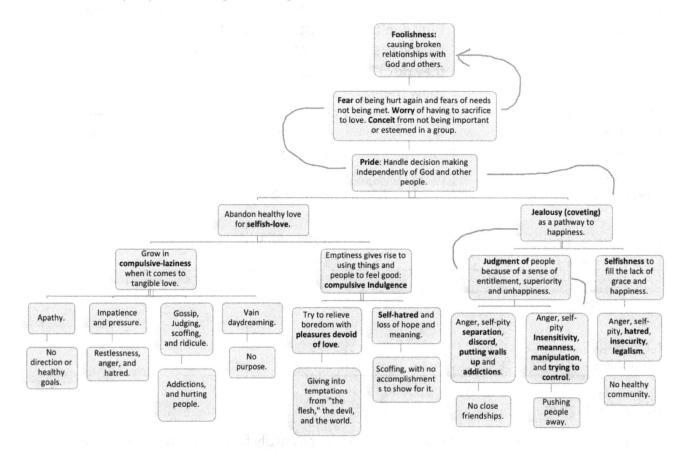

With the corresponding Sin-Anatomy Table below:

Insensitivity	Judging	Jealousy and coveting	Pride	Fear/ Fear/ Conceit	Foolishness
	<=	<=	<=	<=	<= Cause and Effect
Ignore the suffering of others. Write off other people's feelings and destiny as not important or valid.	Me vs. Them. I minimize other people's suffering and not my own.	I want to be cool like others. I covet fairness above all things.	I have a martyr complex. I'm more important than others. I don't care for others if they don't care for me.	Angst because I might be left out of the picture. Afraid I won't belong.	Lies believed: Lying is OK if you get what you want. Peers were unreasonable about what it took to belong. Hated those close to me when they didn't fit into my plans. Feelings are not important.
Did this for years without realizing a way out…					
Confession & Repenting in Faith =>	=>	=>	=>	=>	

Prayer:

Hi Lord Jesus, here I am again processing my emotions. I confess that I ignore the suffering of others. I write off other people's feelings too easily. And often their destiny is not important enough for me to have a more fitting attitude towards. This is sinful. Please forgive me [Done Rene]. I give up these sins with your help through faith in you Jesus.

Lord God, I confess that I still judge people with a "Me vs. Them" mentality thinking their sufferings mean nothing but mine do. Please forgive me [Done Rene]. I give up this mentality and choose to care instead for people through faith and with your help Jesus.

Lord God, I confess that I want to be cool like others and that I covet my brand of fairness at all costs, but I do this all with unhealthy energy and massive blind spots. I give this up with your help through faith in you Jesus; please forgive me [Done Rene]. Thanks Jesus!

Lord God, I confess that I have a selfish martyr complex. I feel I give up so much because of other people visiting their agendas on me. I did this out of fear and weakness. Instead I give up giving up what's important to me with your help Jesus. Lord God, I confess that I see myself as being more important than others, and if they don't care, then I pout and choose to not care for them either. Lord God, I give up these lies that fuel my pride, with your help through faith in you.

Lord God, I confess that I have angst that I will be left out of things and that I won't belong. I felt like I did not belong as a child in South Africa and it was horrible. But you the living God have promised to never leave me nor forsake me. Lord God, I choose to give up these fears through faith in you and I hold onto your love in faith because you are a good God. I choose to fight for what I believe in from now on and for whom I care about and not motivate myself by my fears. I don't have to take a "No" from someone as the final answer. People are often open to compromise. And those who repent and make amends are often very welcome by those they offended.

Lord God, this is all built up from the foolish lies I believed as a child and held onto subconsciously as an adult. Seeing them for the lies they are helps to free me. I give up my jaded views of what makes a relationship work. I choose to believe instead: (a) that lying is not an acceptable building block to building relationships, (b) My peers weren't unreasonable. I gave up too easy in making amends, and (c) Everyone has feelings and I need to respect this. Thank you for loving me Jesus, Father God and Holy Spirit. Amen!

Results: Feel human again. My intuition at navigating relationships is back. Don't feel blindsided. I have love in my heart. I have heartfelt caring within me again because I care for the whole person not just whether they are doing right or wrong.

9.11: Diagnosing And Healing Greed And Selfishness

The belief that we should come first (i.e. having jealousy and envy) translates into doing everything to be first (i.e. having selfishness and greed).

Pride leads to greed for two reasons: prideful people must have more possessions than others do to feel good about themselves; and because fear and self-pity motivate pride insatiably, we never have enough. Until we can process fear and self-pity in a healthy way, it will always be there. When I observe seemingly, to be left out of something, the inclination is to feel jealousy, anger, and to make judgments. But owning and exploring these spiritual diseases through confession and repentance in prayer via Sin-Conduit Structures is a doorway to inner transformation. This way I am able to process my current values, commitments, and thinking behind it all. Therefore, I am able to transition from judgment and self-pity to truth telling by renewing my mind's foundational beliefs, commitments, loyalties and attitudes.

Prayer: Dismantling A Selfish Leadership Approach

The prayer below is recorded chronologically, and not backwards like the others. My hindsight is

20/20 on this one, and it is just too complicated to record in reverse.

We can be selfish in many areas of our lives. Leadership was one such area in my life. Here I was dismantling a multi-sin Sin-Conduit Structure dealing with bad motives and an unhealthy style in leadership. It had the following form below:

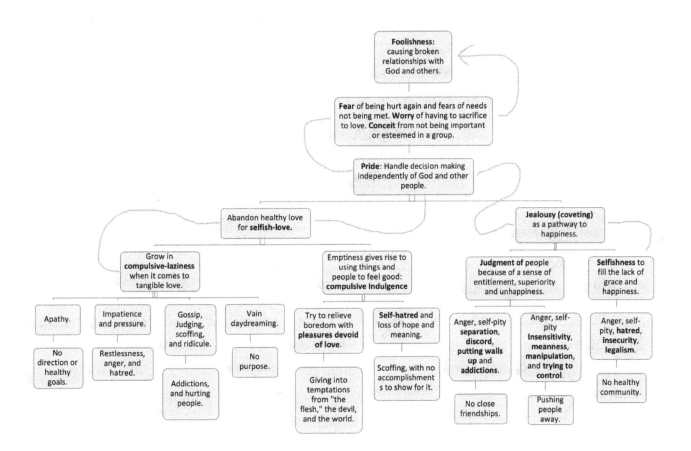

Self-Explanatory Prayer

"Lord God, I confess that as a child I foolishly set my heart on leadership because I wanted to be first, and not to serve other's best interests like you commanded. Please forgive me for this. Thank you. I choose to give this up with your help in faith right now.

Lord God, I confess that I feared not being number one because I felt insecure. I confess my conceit, and self-pity as being tools to further my unhealthy cause of being first. Please forgive me Jesus, and heal my heart, as I can do nothing good without your help. I give up these sins with your help by faith in Jesus.

Lord God, I admit to my pride of wanting things to revolve around me, and using force on others to achieve my legalistic standards of getting my way wherever I am. Please forgive me, a sinner, Lord God. Please heal me too. Thank you. Lord God, I give up this sin-stronghold with your help by faith in Jesus.

Lord God, I confess that I have selfish-love growing out of my pride. I have been tempted to use people to prop up my self-esteem and further my grandiose schemes and opinions of myself. Please forgive and heal me, Lord God. Thank you. Lord God, I give up these sins with your help by faith in Jesus.

Lord God, I confess my sin of compulsive-laziness in wanting to push others with pressure and force so I don't have to do anything and get a false peace out of it. Please forgive me, Lord God. Thank you. I give these sins up with your help through faith in Jesus. Amen.

Lord God, I confess that my pride made me covet being number one more than caring about others. This is selfishness on my part. I saw leadership as more about me and my ways than caring for those I was called to lead. Lord God, I ask you to forgive and heal me of these sins. I give up these sins with your help by faith in Jesus. Thank you. Amen."

Results

I'm more teachable. I'm learning things more quickly. I'm listening to other people more than before. I'm feeling more connected inside and to reality. I'm more tolerant of other people. I'm able to listen to orchestral music after years of not being able to stomach it.

As far as correct thinking is concerned, I'm aiming for altruism and being generous to others just as God relates with us. The key is to love like we have been loved by Jesus. It is as high as we can aim for and is a positive way to replace the negative commands of, "Do not covet," or the mentality of only seeking personal justice and trying to protect my entitlements and rights.

Further Along

When the stronghold of greed and selfishness is broken our freedom still needs to be maintained through grace and truth via wisdom, prayer, connection and submission to God, and faith in Jesus so God can save us from ourselves. Feelings of anger or jealousy ought not be repressed in prayer to God; they need to be owned—not wrestled with or wholly focused on as right or fitting.

We need to commit to generous giving to those in need out of the peace Jesus gives. We need to deal with coveting, envy, and jealousy; and then deal with pride, fear, foolishness, self-pity, and anger— which will bring freedom from greed.

People who focus on or live by their feelings alone will be slaves to those feelings. If we want to completely conquer unwanted strongholds, then we need to change our beliefs through the grace and truth of Jesus Christ; we do this through confession, repentance in prayer, renewing our minds, and aiming to live out Jesus' commands with His help.

If resentment and selfishness go unhealed, then it will warp one's attitudes, intuitions, perspectives, and relationships. This quest for healing and making room for healthy attitudes, desires, and thinking, can be a real fight and a work of labor through prayer.[41] To work out our salvation in fear and trembling means to clean our insides so our relational outsides are clean too. Praying through blockages, receiving the promises of God, and resisting the devil's attempts to cause confusion and immobilization is key. We should deal with those areas that confuse us and those that have no obvious solution. There are ways through and out of challenges—maybe not pleasant ways, but noble ones. Let's reason together with God, and He will anoint our thinking when we seek Him with all our hearts. Knowing His voice is essential for breakthroughs.

When I get free in this or any area, then I need to move back to focusing on what Jesus is saying to me next, and continue to let Him save me through my trust in Him. Principles and truths have their limitations, only the Divine Principle (Jesus) is enough. I choose to follow Him alone.

9.12: Diagnosing And Healing Judgments And Jealousy

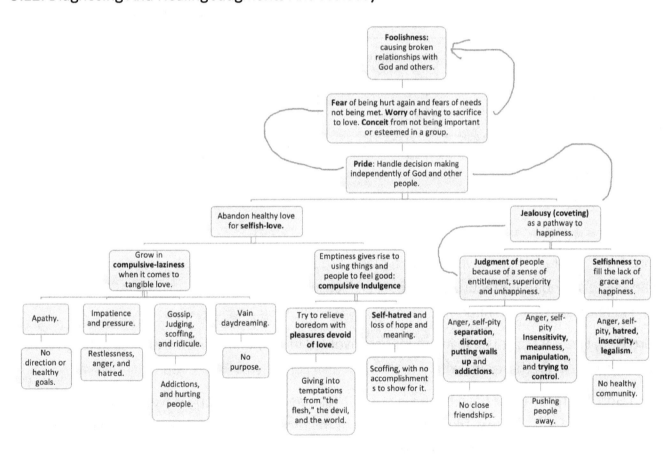

The Sin-Conduit Structure above has the following Sin-Anatomy Table, and when prayed through corrected my history of blaming and judging people in the context of my jealousy, doing

---

[41] As far as my struggle to know what healthy love and humility look like cf. my books called: *Exploring Faith, Hope & Love,* and *Contrasting Humility and Pride.*

chores and work requests as I relate in chapter 8.2. It also struck a blow to my disliking work and my compulsive-laziness:

Self-pity	Judging	Jealousy	Pride	Fear	Foolishness
	<=	<=	<=	<=	<= Cause and Effect
Go to a place of dark self-absorbed self-pity instead of going the extra mile and celebrating grace and the gift of giving to others.	Critical of those who create work for me, or ask me to do projects. I have shown such immaturity in this matter or context most of my life.	Jealous of people who don't have to do chores. Jealous of brother and sister in this matter when growing up.	I'm committed to being first in so many contexts in my life. Everything should revolve around me.	Fear of having to give up pleasurable time spent on my own pursuits in order to give sacrificial love when asked. Fear of being singled out repeatedly to do work.	Not forgiving Dad for in my eyes unfairly delegating work duties when I was a child and was singled out to work in the garden by myself.
I lost out so often in not being unselfish thereby not finding meaning and purpose...					
Confession & Repenting in Faith =>	=>	=>	=>	=>	

Prayer

Lord God, I confess that I have gone to a place of dark, self-absorbed self-pity, desperately wanting to say no to perfectly good requests. Please forgive me. I give up doing this with your help in faith Lord Jesus. Thank you.

Lord God, I confess that I have judged those involved in very immature ways. Please forgive me. I choose to give up these sins with your help in faith Lord Jesus. Thank you.

Lord God, I confess that I have been jealous of those people who don't have the same obligations as I do. I confess that I was jealous of my brother and sister when I was younger too. Please forgive me. I give up my jealousy with your help in faith. Thank you.

I confess that I still struggle to not be the center of the universe expecting everyone to cater to my whims. Please forgive me. I give up this pride with your help in faith Lord Jesus. Thank you.

I confess I have the fear of being singled out when it comes to doing work or projects as I don't want to give up pleasurable activities in the face of sacrificial calls to love. Please forgive me. I give up these fears with your help through faith in you Jesus. Thank you.

Lord God, I confess that I have never forgiven my Dad for his delegating of chores in what seemed to me at the time as unfair. Please forgive me. I forgive him now with your help in faith, giving up all my judgments against him. Thank you and amen.

9.13: Malicious Judgments

Judging also occurs when one thinks horrible things about another person. Often the bad things we think are not verifiable. But they are so bad that we rationalize it with our self-righteous anger over some trespass committed by the person we are judging. This kind of judging believes the utter worst about people. It too needs to be confessed and repented from in prayer where relevant sin-conduits exist that contain the judgments. When we process this kind of judgment, then we become patient people.

10 Summarizing How I Dismantle The Tree Of Knowledge Of Good And Evil Within My Life

Working out the connections between the tree's building blocks by just analyzing concepts (without prayer and God) can lead to burdens, emptiness, and a lack of grace to change. In becoming aware of the connections in "the tree of knowledge of good and evil," it is best to look at our bad fruit and ask what foolish beliefs, judgments, anger, sin and possible self-pity, causes them to grow. We also have to ask the Holy Spirit which lies keep the tree structure intact through foolishness and fears; and construct Sin-Anatomy Tables as the Holy Spirit speaks to us in our thoughts. Once the connections are understood it is time to dismantle them through strategic prayer that allows for the process of renewing our minds. We construct detailed Sin-Anatomy Tables to keep the guessing and frustration to a minimum; it helps us to find and dismantle the real motivations, roots, and powers in our sin strongholds more quickly—and we eventually find freedom to love people more deeply.

The growth of "the tree of the knowledge of good and evil" works in such a manner that creates distance between us and God. We begin to doubt, question, and disbelieve God's promise to be with us, care for us, and bless us. When Adam and Eve sinned in the Garden of Eden, they did not know God's forgiveness, and started to blame whomever or whatever was convenient because they felt lost. They had fears to deal with. "The tree of knowledge of good and evil" came between them and God just like it does with us and God. When we are forgiven, then we have peace with God, and His peace rests in our hearts. The devil does everything he can to plant lies in our minds to rob us of this peace. When dealing with broken relationships, forgiveness helps to mend our hurts and lift our burdens.

When using anger and self-pity to get our way, we are saying no to loving others because everything is geared to selfishness. Choosing love and altruism in the place of anger and self-pity are the keys to softening the heart, creating warmth and no longer being the center of our own universe.

Living a superficial life where there are no roots, no enduring values, and no commitments to caring for people is a result of fear, conceit, and self-pity. The fear comes because there is little trust: no real knowledge of genuine love, no understanding that people care, and no motivation for living for a higher purpose. When problems are revealed below the surface, embarrassment, fear of rejection, denial, and donning masks become the order of the day.

Sometimes praying to uproot pride does not work because the spiritual malady does have other roots that must be dealt with too. For instance, I realized that a wall often came up in me, pushing others away, when the healthy thing to do was to care for and feel other people's pains, frustrations and struggles. Pride was involved but it wasn't the mother lode in this context, and confessing only pride didn't heal the wound of insensitivity. However, confessing and repenting in prayer from the unwillingness to trust, the insensitivity to not care or feel for others, and to having an arrogant attitude—and then asking God for forgiveness and healing in faith through grace did help.

Choosing to care for people and to willingly dispense grace—as far as the Golden Rule is concerned, and out of the peace God puts into my heart—helps break the walls I have erected to vainly protect me against rejection. Grace is never stagnant. It flows into me and out of me when I relate to others in healthy ways.

Sometimes we think we have exhausted praying about the vices in "the tree of knowledge of good and evil" and feel stuck. I have found it has to do with nine things:

1. Not accepting God's will for our lives (i.e. not accepting that we are perfectly imperfect, and shit happens).
2. Ignoring real or false guilt.
3. Caring more about one's knowledge of spiritual things than *actually* caring about and loving people practically.
4. Not submitting to God and resisting the devil.
5. Not having processed uncomfortable emotions and not using "I" statements to renew the mind.
6. Blaming, attacking, or judging God and others; and pursuing anger, pressure, and self-pity as means to getting what we want.
7. Not going deeper into the healing process in prayer with Jesus' help.
8. Not living in the present by embracing and celebrating God's grace.
9. Praying in faith but ending with unbelief in the same prayer (i.e. being double minded).

Having certain feelings doesn't always mean our thinking is justified, natural, and healthy just because those feelings resonate with us. Thoughts determine feelings. Therefore we reject inappropriate, negative, callous beliefs and thinking. And we replace them with truthful, positive, and loving thoughts and beliefs. It does not normally work the other way around. However, we can have negative attitudes that are so sour, bitter, and judgmental that they just unwantedly spout out of our hearts. This needs to be prayed through with gentle, genuine, honest, strategic prayers; when we have enough clarity of mind so we can sort through our confusion and emotions, and when the memories are fresh enough.

When we are renewing our minds we will encounter plenty of confusion.[42] Because we might be torn between our old beliefs and thinking and the light of Jesus in our consciences, we need to be patient and persistent and hold onto Jesus' grace and truths (His promises, His presence, His

---

[42] I have written about topics that have confused me in the books: *Exploring Faith, Hope & Love* and *Contrasting Humility and Pride.*

teachings, and His example). We need to ask Him for direction and believe He will provide.

So how do we overcome our reluctance to love because of judgments that put us in danger of not carrying out the Golden Rule? Through grace, unconditional love or love without conditions.

What focus ought we to have in order to make love real to those we meet daily? How do we love them unconditionally and further dismantle our strongholds of sin? Put another way how are we: "to love without conditions" the people in our lives?

It is helpful to ask what sorts of conditions exist that keep us from loving unconditionally the people in our lives? There are many, but the "Do they deserve my love?" is the strongest condition I can think of that stops us from loving people. It is often tied to revenge or "An eye for an eye, and a tooth for a tooth"[43] mentality. The idea being that people ought to get what they deserve because it is only fair.

When I start to wrestle with and take offence at the boundary violations or hurts others have visited on me when I look for reasons to love, then this path can easily lead towards judging, self-pity, anger, resentments, unkindness and a lack of love if I'm not careful.

A quick and easy way to put such judging to death is to ask myself: "Do I want to be gracious to the guilty party?" Or ask: "Do I want to love them unconditionally?" If I answer yes to these questions, then the judging shackles fall to the ground as grace flows into me enabling me to do an act of love with God's grace. That touches the life of someone I was tempted to formerly treat like an enemy instead.

This is not done through minimizing what the guilty party did or didn't do, but it is done because we know about and experience God's grace or unconditional love each day. And we want God's grace for everyone not just ourselves. God's love inspires us to love unconditionally. The fewer sin strongholds in our lives the stronger and more likely this strategy is going to help bear love.

There are many strongholds against love besides judging. Such as compulsive laziness, jealousy, wanting things to be fair, self-pity, anger, conceit, pride, and using people to get what we want to mention a few. When such blocks are dealt with then love can and will blossom more fully.

The only way to growing in love involves repenting in wise, genuine and caring ways. When we get unhealthy stuff that is sinful, negative, mean, intolerant, jealous, and manipulative triggered within us (while interacting with a person) then such attitudes are doorways to change when we know how to pray.

Prayer is so important to maintain a close relationship with God, and replace an unhealthy view of God with a merciful, caring, kind, and loving experience of God. Challenging sour attitudes

---

[43] Cf. Exodus 21:24

towards God can be done by reading about Jesus in the Gospels and realizing He reflects the likeness of God the Father. The gentle words of Jesus inspire us to turn away from our angry and sour attitudes and beliefs, as we trust His forgiveness, grace, truth, compassion, wisdom, plans, actions, and invitations.

There are many good books on how to cultivate healthy two-way prayer such as those written by Brad Jersak and Mark Virkler. They can help to clear up our confusion, demonstrate how to walk through confusion into the light, or guide us to have more inward clarity. Prayer is not just about petitions, but about communion, hearing each other, and touching God.

I want to stress that when we pray, as outlined in this book and in certain contexts that seem difficult, then it is a healthy idea to repeatedly go deeper when crafting prayers the Holy Spirit helps us to pray. We need to patiently search for genuine love.

11 Applying The Methodology Learned To Some Examples In My Personal Life

As you may realize by now, each person's personal "tree of knowledge of good and evil" is different; it depends on the situations encountered, the resulting bad decisions, foolish loyalties, and bad commitments made, and the lies believed.

I will share six examples of how God helped me to dismantle some strongholds found in my personal "tree of knowledge of good and evil" within. I believe that the methodology and strategies found in this book can help people who struggle with the same difficulties I found in my heart—and maybe even struggles not talked about in this book, but spoken about in the Bible too.

The strategy is simple: when I am aware of weakness or compulsive sins in my life (those things that go against loving God, people and ourselves), I find my way through the parts of "the tree of Knowledge of good and evil" diagram that speak most clearly to my situation and history; I then begin to speak to God about the connections and ask Him to give me awareness and insight to flesh out the connections in my personal life of sin; finally I write down my prayerful conversation and the lies I believed using Sin-Anatomy Tables, and work through the issues in prayer with God until the structure is permanently dismantled. Often there are multiple roots per stronghold so praying things from different angles as the Holy Spirit leads—asking, searching, knocking on doors, not just waiting around or giving up—will eventually bring the truth and grace that opens up freedom.

Dealing with your fears and broken relationships are usually the final steps to healing, and it means repenting from any sins that helped cause the broken relationships and dealing with the lies and resentments I believe or hold onto.

11.1: Tackling Insensitivity

The Situation

I'm *really* hard on others. That means I'm insensitive, mean, and manipulative when what I covet won't come my way. Most of the time I'm a really kind person, but when I *really* want something badly, then my fear and pride triggers my war chest of judgment and being hard on others so that I will somehow get my way. The fact is I'm hard on others because I'm hard on myself (in this context but not in all contexts). The bad fruit is that I end up acting like a jerk and pushing people away.

How do I deal with it so it doesn't reoccur anymore, and how do I become more gentle and patient?

Following the dark, arrowed line or Sin-Conduit Structure, in the "tree of knowledge of good and evil" diagram below, I will show how I prayed through the different areas of this particular relational situation:

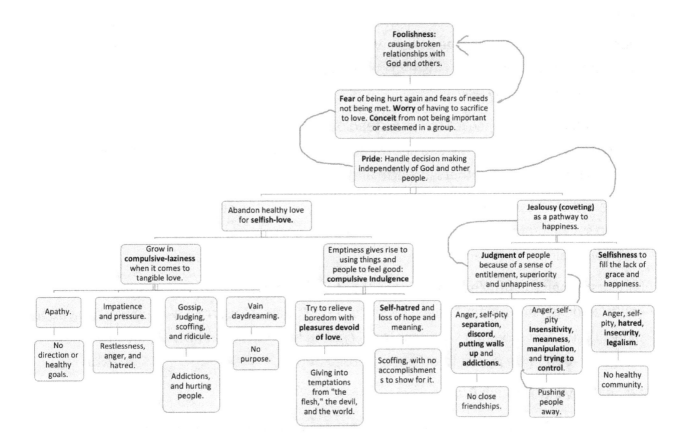

Finding My Bearings

First, I need to ask God for wisdom and ask the Holy Spirit for healing. Then I start processing the situation by recounting the emotions , facts, and memories relating to the baggage or struggles I have. Then I choose to talk with God about it; I confess the details, conflicts, confusion, difficulty, sins, and bad attitudes I have related to the area I'm dealing with. I must find some clean energy, some humility, or some purity somewhere in my heart and mind which I can pray from. And I choose to do so with a caring mindset, so that I eventually get to a place of not attacking or judging God and others.

Prayer

"Lord God, I admit and confess that I am hard on people, as far as my attitudes go. I have a dark, mean energy within me when things don't go my way. I know all this blackness is found in my war chest to get my way in the most jerk-like fashion possible.

Lord Jesus, I have depended on this war chest in the cavity of my heart, as my energy in getting people to comply with my wishes, even though I hide this darkness really well most of the time. It is self-pity and anger geared to get my way. I admit that the self-pity and angry pressure use to have a prominent place in my heart, but I don't need it anymore. I choose to welcome the Holy Spirit in my heart instead, to submit to Him, and resist the devil.

I admit that I impatiently judge others who are in my way. With your help Jesus, I give up saying no to this energy, and I instead choose to give up my judgments and forceful manipulation to get my way.

I confess that I jealousy covet things instead of being generous. With your help Jesus, I give up saying no to this, and I instead choose to give up coveting things for myself alone when it ought to be shared with others in warm and good-natured ways.

I confess that I have plenty of pride—that I see myself as the center of the whole universe. I give up saying no to agreeing with this compulsive energy, and instead I choose to give it up with your help through faith Jesus.

Lord Jesus, I give up my fears of going without and of being second. I give up these fears as you provide generously for me and others so I don't have to worry. I give up worrying about things I can't and shouldn't try to control. I choose to be wiser on how I set my heart on things so I don't give power to others and lose control."

Renewing the Mind Through Prayer

Lord God, I felt self-pity, anger, bitterness, hatred, and meanness after I felt the wound of rejection as a child in school. I focus a lot of that energy on myself, and it still hurts to this day.

Lord God, I went into a rebellious mode, a conformity mode, and a legalistic mode all fused together in a horrible mess. It was all out of fear—fears of missing out. I give up that fear now with your grace, Jesus; I give up the mixture of rebellion, conformity, and legalism within me because they are empty cisterns. You are with me Jesus: walking with me, wanting my healing, being my peace, salvation, life, joy and consolation.

So this is my stronghold of fear; fear of missing out: on having happiness, on being first, on having instant peace or gratification, on having the easy way, on being on the inside, on having loyalty, on being in covenant, on having solidarity, and on unending friendship bliss. Fear and a demanding nature motivates it all out of my pride and suggests all the wrong ways to attain these things.

Either I'm very good at lying to myself or I'm very foolish for believing the devil's lies in this context. Satan, I reject your lies that I'll miss out on things unless I act out of my "sin nature." I accept my sin nature for what it is, but I don't need it right now; Jesus, I give this up with your help through faith. Because Jesus is sufficient with grace upon grace. Amen.

This led to the following two truths that liberated me a little while later:

1. How do I stand up and ask for something with flexibility? Not rigidly, darkly, or in an ugly, demanding, have to have it way without compromise. Humility gives others a choice in the matter and empowers them without giving the impression that they have to meet my requests. This frees me and others to laugh and love in freedom instead of compulsively demanding things for selfish reasons.
2. I must become able to accept the healthy no's from others. This helps to cure my use of self-pity and anger to get my way, and helps me to start respecting and loving people instead.

Next, I prayed to give up the strongholds of inflexibility and refusing to accept no in my requests.

But all of this does not go far enough. I needed to give up my judgment of (i.e. wrongly blaming) my peers and myself for allowing the hurt to be inflicted on me in grade school:

"Lord God, I give up my judgment against my peers, in their youth and as adults. And I forgive myself now with your help. I choose to love them and myself from now on with your grace and truth. Thank you Jesus for forgiving me my resentments, hatred, and meanness directed towards all the people I wanted things from, and for not having the proper respect for them."

That is how I prayed through one portion of "the tree of knowledge of good and evil" within me to bring healing. Notice how it deals with my history, the wound, understanding the lies I believed, telling Satan I reject his lies, and repenting in prayer from it all. I also needed to forgive and assert that Jesus is generous and sufficient in providing all the peace I need because He is always with me.

Going Deeper In Prayer

God told me that I still hated myself and my South African peers even after forgiving them and myself over and over. This precipitated looking at the following Sin-Conduit Structure:

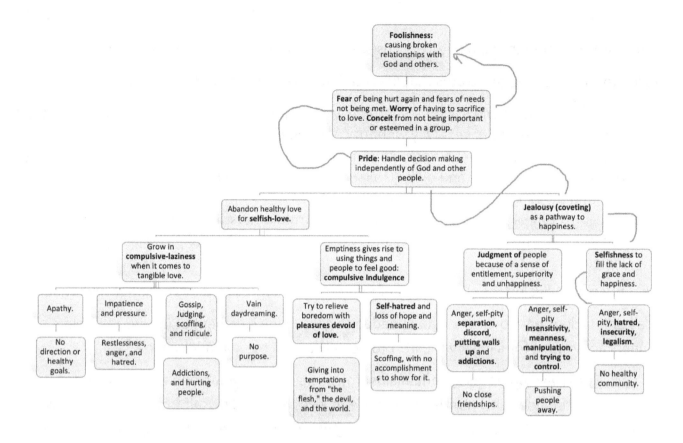

With the corresponding Sin-Anatomy Table:

Hatred	Selfishness	Coveting	Pride	Fear	Foolishness
	<=	<=	<=	<=	<= Cause and Effect
Hate myself and my SA peers, because I feel unloved and am pushing people away. A self fulfilling prophecy.	First and foremost I must make sure I'm looked after, and am number one before anyone else. Thereby pushing people away.	Covet being number one, having friends, and set my heart on being a nice person so people will like me.	I am the center of the universe. I get to decide what I live by- no one else; not even God.	Motivated by fear of being hurt again.	I believed the lie that I'm unloveable, that no body loves me; not even God.
Generally I have low self-esteem, and I don't even respect myself....					
Confession & Repenting in Faith =>	=>	=>	=>	=>	

Prayer

"Lord God, I confess that after all these years I still hate myself and those I felt were responsible for my implosion. I give up doing this with your help Jesus. This hatred comes from my selfishness that says, "I'm going to look after myself first, before anyone else in my life," thereby pushing everyone away—even you my God. Lord God, I give up this commitment with your help through faith in you.

I admit that my selfishness comes from coveting being number one and being a nice person so people will like me; the idea being that they will like me because I'm nice and not because I'm a human made in God's image. But choosing to be number one pushes people away, so I end up thinking there is something wrong with me. Because I don't let others become close to me or allow them to love me I hate myself more. I give this up, with your help Lord Jesus, by faith. This strategy comes from my pride that says I get to choose what I live by not anyone else—not even God. Lord God, I'm sorry. I motivate myself by fear of being hurt again. I give this up with your help Lord Jesus, by faith in you. Lord God, this comes from believing the lie that I'm unlovable, and nobody loves me. I give up this lie. And I declare that you the Living God love me, and I therefore choose to love myself fully too. Thank you for forgiving and healing me, Lord Jesus. Amen."

When people don't fully love themselves or fully respect themselves, then there are sometimes others who will pick-up on this and despise this about them. They may care for them but find it intolerable that such persons are weak and unloving of themselves.

We can be hard on ourselves in one context, and soft on ourselves in other contexts. The above example deals with the former, the next one deals with latter.

11.2: Tackling Pride

To work through the Tree Diagram you do not have to start right at the bottom. Often we can be stuck in a certain part of "the tree of knowledge of good and evil" within, and bear obsessive and compulsive fruit there too. Here is one example:

The situation

I realized that when I judged people I did so in a way where I was much harder on them than I was on myself. This part of the tree has malice formed out of a mixture of pride and blindness.

Getting One's Bearings

Below is "the tree of knowledge of good and evil" diagram and in order to pray it I follow the Sin-Conduit Structure:

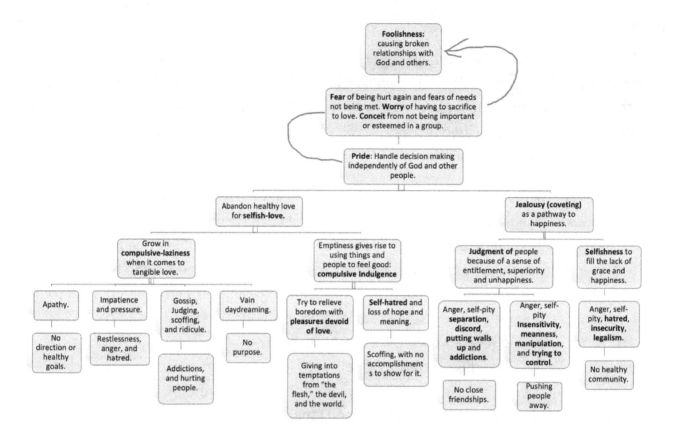

Prayer

"Lord Jesus, I admit that I have lots of pride in this context. It is lethal. I *actually* want my "pound of flesh" from these people for what they have done. And in my pride, I have judged myself to be better than them just like in the parable of the unmerciful servant. I give this up with your help, through faith in you Lord Jesus, and I choose to celebrate life, love, and tolerance in my relationships instead. I admit that I have seen people as worthy of my wrath, revenge, and rejection not realizing I'm no better than anyone else either.

Lord God, what fears are behind this?

I fear not getting what I think I am owed, I deserve, or I have a claim to. I fear because I have chosen to not trust people. I have a history of being skeptical of the goodness of others.

Lord God, I give up this fear here and now. Please help me to see the goodness in others and to appeal to their nobility; and not to use what I see as their guilt and shame to pressure and force things from them that I desire. Thank you, Jesus.

I admit that behind this fear is rejection. I have been rejected so often and never processed any of it in healthy ways. Here and now, I choose to forgive those people who have hurt me through rejection over my lifetime.

I admit that because I feel powerless in this context that I default to an attitude of self-pity, anger, and despair. I confess this as wrong and give up my self-pity and anger as tools to get what I want. I choose instead to love the people who trigger my reactions in this context.

Lord God, I thirst for your Holy Spirit, I hunger for your presence, and I rest in your love. Please help me to renew my mind with your truth so that I will know how good and pleasing your will is. I submit to your will. I renounce the devil and all his empty promises and lies.

Jesus, you are sufficient with grace and truth because you never run from a fight; you are my constant companion, my real peace, and my consolation. Amen."

Going Deeper in Prayer

"Lord God, I confess my pride in these forms of thinking: that I always know better than others (because they are stupid and I am more intelligent); that I am most important and others must come last at all costs; and that no one is going to 'pull one over' on me. I am sorry and ask for your forgiveness and healing receiving them deeply within me. Thank you, Jesus.

Dear God, in faith and with your help, I give up saying no to my pride. I instead renew my mind. I give up the sinful attitudes of thinking I'm most important, I must not come last, and I'm not gullible. I give up the corresponding belief that others need to come last and I must be first, and that others need to live according to my values, expectations, and morality. I give up all the patterns of thoughts, speech, and behaviors that I have used in the past up to the present. Please help me to renew my mind, heart, and behaviors in this area. Thank you, Jesus.

Lord Jesus I give up self-righteously saying no to the sin of cowardice, of choosing to play it safe, and of not taking chances; I give these up and ask for your help instead. I give up the lies that if there is not enough for everyone then I need to do everything in my power to get what is mine. Lord God, I confess my fears: of not getting what others may have, of not having or losing friends, and of being left behind when events take place. Lord God I give up these fears and sins with your help, and I choose to renew my mind with commonsense truths along with your truths. Please help me to practice humility instead of my pride. Lord God, you deserve all the glory, because you are the source of all good things. Thank you for making us conduits of your grace. Amen.

11.3: Tackling The Tendency To Push People Away

The Situation

The situation is the same as the last example of judging others harshly. Often when the hurt goes *really* deep we need to go deeper in prayer, since there are multiple "sin-conduits" that need to be dealt with from various angles. I deal with more layers in this example.

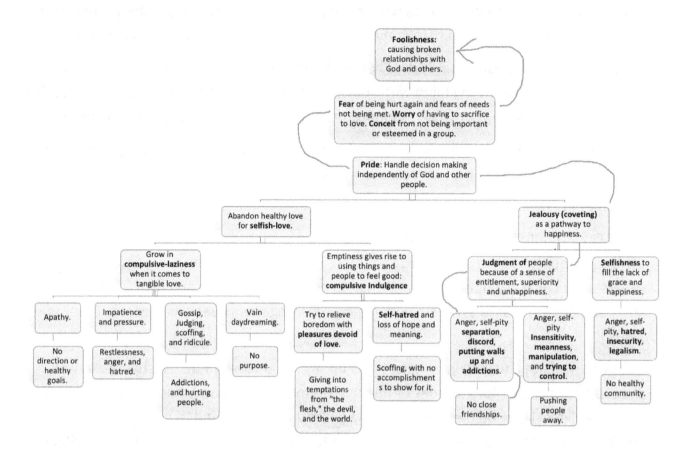

Prayer

"Lord God, I'm sorry for pushing people away and refusing to connect with them in caring ways. I commit to giving this up, through faith in you Lord Jesus, and caring for people from now on with your grace and truth.

Lord God, I admit that a wall of insensitivity rises within me that shows carnal energy—when my fear-induced, broken, moral compass sees violations of any rule or law. Lord Jesus, I choose to lower this wall, recalibrate my expectations, and renew my compass with your truth, light, and healing. Mercy triumphs over judgment, retribution, and revenge. Kindness leads to change—not meanness.

I have judged others as convenient scapegoats. I search for goodness within but my mind conjures up mostly mean judgments, condemnation, malice and a desire to hurt certain people. Through faith in you Jesus, I give up both condemning others who are made in your image and hurting people because of my hurt. I choose the love and forgiveness that comes from you the source of all goodness, Lord God. Your word says don't pay back evil with evil, and so I give this up with your help through faith.

I have envied the strong and have committed to being seen as strong no matter what the consequences are. I give this up now through faith in you Lord Jesus. I choose to be despised, rejected, hated, and uncared for so long as I'm doing your will—loving you the Living God and my neighbor as myself.

Lord God, I have legalistically conformed to the supposed thinking and actions of those who rejected me as a child. They seemed in control, strong, popular, and healthier than those they ridiculed, hurt, hated, and judged. I wrongfully wanted what they had, and I was willing to pay the price to belong. I give this up right now, in faith and with your help Lord Jesus, based on the blood that you shed on the cross for each of us. Thank you.

Lord God, I admit I have done all of this out of being hurt and out of the fear of being hurt again. I give up this fear, through faith in you the living God, and ask that you heal me from this broken structure within. Therefore, I forgive them from my heart, choosing to love the weak and the strong as you do Jesus.

Holy Trinity, I invite you into my life more fully. I choose to live out the Golden Rule, to lower my walls, and to love those I'm called to care about. Thank you for forgiving me, Father God. Thank you for not leaving me to my own devices and pouring your grace into my heart and life.

Lord God, please help me to renew my mind with your truth inwardly, and my relationships outwardly. I await your truth, seek your will, and reject the devil, his lies and his empty promises. I pray all of this in Jesus' name. Amen."

Renewing My Mind

Lord God, in the past I tried to avoid hurt by pretending I was okay, putting up walls, and trying to join those who proudly wielded power. But it did not work. In trying to save my life I lost it—along with the rich communion you offer, and relationship with my fellow man. I now choose to embrace hurt, because truth, love, justice, honor, respect, and caring for people are the healthier goals. When I am weak in the world's eyes, then I am strong in God's eyes. And your grace is sufficient, Lord Jesus. Lord God, I ask for the gift of courage to replace my cowardice, conceit, and pride. Thank you. Amen.

Summary

It is important to not copy the exact ideas and requests made in the above prayers when praying your own prayers. Leave room for your own unique, personality, story, and history, for the leading of the Holy Spirit, and for making the effort to dig into your own heart and mind for your own truth. Get your own bearings so you can follow Jesus into the light. When we undertake to humble ourselves before God, then He grants His empowering presence and the desired freedom eventually comes.

11.4: Dealing With Deception And An Unwanted Smile

Situation

I took a risk and lost a gamble in grade school when I tried to be accepted by my peers by lying, but I got rejected instead. I have had unwanted consequences happen, in part because of my reactions in childhood, that have wreaked havoc on my spiritual life for 40-plus years. I prayed into this area somewhat, but there was still a festering wound. So I needed to go deeper in prayer. I found out in difficult ways that not contritely confessing and repenting of my lying to my peers was at the bottom of it all; it was the cause of me having "the tree of knowledge of good and evil" within me eat up so much of my healthy interior and relational life. It had the following Sin-Conduit Structure:

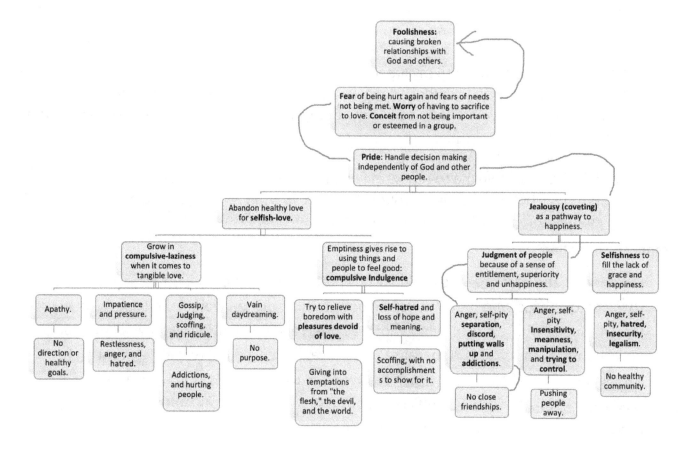

Prayer

"Lord God, I confess that I hurt so much, and I set walls and put on masks to not let others get close to me because fear of being hurt keeps them there. I said no to ever being hurt again, but I give this up with your help Jesus, and choose to navigate my relationships without guarantees that I won't be hurt again. I can do all things through you, Jesus Christ, who strengthens me.

I admit I became black inside: hollow, cold, dark and starved for love. I give this up in faith and with your help, Lord Jesus. I invite your warmth, presence, and authority into the dark rooms of my heart. You are most welcome Holy Trinity.

In faith and with your help Jesus, I give up my judgments, hatred, anger and pressure directed at myself and my enemies. Please heal my heart Jesus. Thank you so much for your promises, truth, and healing.

Lord God, I confess that I have been jealous of my peers' friendships, relationships, and seeming blissful happiness, which I did not have because of my inner-walls of protection. I give up saying no to my jealousy and instead give up this jealousy, with your help Jesus and through faith. Thank you.

I put so much pressure on myself to belong, to have the perfect self-image, to be strong, and to hide my broken heart. None of this gave me what I wanted: connection, belonging, peace, hope, and happiness. Lord God, I give up putting this pressure on myself, with your help. I embrace your breath of life, grace, hope, truth, and presence from now on. I give up the fear of being hurt again, with your help. And I embrace your wisdom, love, and care for me instead. Thank you.

Lord God, I forgive myself for my pride, independence, and foolishness. I give up my judgments against my peers; they are who they are, with no more judgment from me. Amen."

Revelations

"I can't save myself through lies, through my own energy, or through my pride. I can't save myself with deception, motivated by fears, and leaving my hurts unhealed. With your help Lord Jesus, I give up my self-righteous attempts, proud struggles, carnal energy, and rigid commitments to save myself by wearing a mask, that only ever ended up with me hurting people in my attempt to not be hurt. I pray all of this admitting my guilt and intellectually and emotionally receive your forgiveness and healing.

Wearing a mask is a necessity when there is fear, unless one knows and experiences caring, gentleness, and deep unconditional love. So if I don't want a mask, then I must give up the fear and embrace God—the love that can't be shaken. But how do I do this? I confront my history of fears inspired in some cases by being hurt so badly. And I confront the false beliefs behind them so they lose their power. The masks are slowly coming off, as I process in prayer all the situations where I wore it as my protection or salvation. Jesus, you are my real salvation. Amen."

Confronting My Fears

There are four categories of fears: rejection, abandonment, confrontation, and death. As stated previously, we need to process and confront them by attacking the beliefs behind them: in prayer, with humble truth, preferably by writing them out and then speaking them out loud. We simply list the fears, we give them up in faith, and we affirm commonsense wisdom and biblical truth and promises about love through prayer and relationship with God. In doing this we will become less fear motivated and more love motivated. Everyone will have their own lists. Here are a few of mine:

1. **I fear being without a mask**. "Lord Jesus, I know that the mask is an idol that keeps me from real, wholesome, warm, caring, and loving salvation. To give it up completely, with your help through faith, I need to redirect and give my fear to you, as your perfect love casts out all fear. I do this now asking you to fill me with your love."

2. **They saw through my facade and that put fear into me**. "Lord Jesus, with your help through faith, I give up this fear of being seen when I'm trying to hide who I am. I'm a poor actor and an even worse liar. I have a "sin nature" and your grace Jesus is more than sufficient."

3. **I fear people.** "Lord Jesus, with your help through faith, I give up my fear of people. Almighty God, I choose to be courageous instead through your Holy Spirit in me."

4. **I fear those close to me.** "Lord Jesus, with your help through faith, I give up my fears of honesty, intimacy, and vulnerability in my relating style. I choose instead to be honest—but not anal—caring, fun, humorous, and playful with your loving help."

5. **I fear being hurt.** "Lord God, hurt is a part of life. With your help through faith, I accept that I will be hurt at times, but I choose to navigate that hurt with your love, your caring, and your example Lord Jesus. Nothing is impossible for you the Living God."

6. **I fear screwing up.** "Perfect love casts out all fear. I walk by faith and not sight. I accept and expect to screw up every now and then, but I choose to handle it with your grace Lord Jesus. I'm perfectly imperfect. Lord Jesus, with your help through faith, I choose to give up my fear of screwing up. Fear does not save, but love saves. Fear is negative, whereas faith, love and hope are positive."

7. **I fear being found out again.** "Lord God, here I am. You know everything about me. You who are most powerful choose to care for me and love me anyways, and so what can others do against me when you are for me?"

A Revelation a Few Weeks Later

For so long, I have seen reality through the lens of "us vs. them," and these past two-weeks God has kindly removed that lens. Last night at bible study, I realized that reality isn't "we are good" and "they are bad," which was my subconscious belief that kept me from loving others more fully and helped keep my "walls" up all the time.

I read my friend Mark's sermon that triggered the need to examine this topic: God is love, and if anything, the only "us vs. them" there could be is God against us all—but His love has bridged the gap. Thank you, Lord God. There is "us and them," but not "us vs. them." Other people are not our enemies, but the devil is. The "we are better" vs. "they are worse" can be in our subconscious and even embedded in our closest relationships. Each instance needs to be uncovered, confessed, and repented from in prayer for it to lose its power. Another attitude of "we are intelligent" vs. "they are stupid" can also be in play. Blanketed prayers won't budge this. We needed to get specific and deal with whatever it grows from for freedom and love to grow in its place.

The way of peace is to war against evil within each of us; not war against the people themselves. And our weapon is to love people more deeply and powerfully through God's grace rather than self-righteously by ourselves.

I came to rely on the truth that "the line between good and evil goes through our hearts and not between people and people groups" heavily but I eventually realized that I needed to go deeper. I realized that I really wanted looking back for God to tell me that I was a good person and did not need to go over to the dark side when I was a child in South Africa when my peers had rejected me. God surprised me by telling it to me in the present and I felt healthier, more centered, stable and at peace as I embraced it. Choosing the correct identity helps to determine our actions.

The Meaning of a Dream

This coincides with the following dream God gave me awhile back: I dreamt that I had this old worn out clutch pencil, like the one I used in university that I tried to make functional again with tape. I was offered a brand new pen to write with, but I rejected it because I thought I knew what I was doing trying to fix the old, broken one. Near the end of the dream, I was told that the "free West was at war with the Communists," and I smugly told myself it would be easily won and I could handle it myself.

I prayed into this night vision recognizing that God was offering me something new. I was quick to reject it within the dream, but while awake I decided to actively pursue the new pen and to sort out the meaning of the war talked about in the dream.

The broken pencil could symbolize that my old, tree life has been broken, and that I needed to give it up completely; and instead of refusing the new pen, which symbolizes new life, I need to accept it. This is what God was inviting me to.

The talk about the "free West" vs. "Communism" I'd later realize was an "us vs. them" or "me vs. them" mentality that I tenaciously held onto for decades. This thinking kept others from getting close to me, kept me from not connecting deeply with others, and kept me from deeply loving the people in my life. I was either loyal to, or an enemy to: certain labels, camps, sects, denominations, traditions, and types. I had difficulty wholeheartedly affirming the good in people I judged with the "wrong designation" no matter how much I wanted to love and connect with them.

I was prevented from fully loving because of this mentality. I therefore chose to focus my prayer life in this area by giving up this "us vs. them" mentality. And I found such peace enter into my life along with the ability to connect with and not habitually judge people like I did before. I felt connected with my true self and others for the first time in many decades. And my "walls" came down too.

"Thank you, Jesus, for the dream. I now understand that you see all things, and you are kind, caring, and gracious to all."

More Revelations

1. I realized that I had been embarrassed about my own positions on a wide variety of topics, because I believed I might be rejected in voicing my beliefs, opinions, convictions, and desires. As a result I would show a huge smile when confronted, as my way to cope with my embarrassment.

2. I also realized that I wanted to control people's opinions of me all the time. This was an impossible task. Because I couldn't, I was again embarrassed and smiled a ridiculously insane smile because I was not in control. Giving up this foolish expectation in prayer by replacing it with humble commonsense truth helped to further set me free from my conceit.

3. Because I let go of my "us vs. them" mentality, my insecurity and fear that God might somehow love some people more than others was dealt a death blow. I knew that if God somehow loved some people more than others then I could not love Him because of my jealousy. But then I realized that God is perfect love, and if He loved someone less than He was capable of, then there was room for His improvement! But God needs no improvement. So, He loves me and everyone no less than any other. This realization brought back my joy of God's salvation, and lifted me up in my ability to love more deeply.

More Prayer Required

Sane people want to love everyone deeply. But when there is a history of war, conflict, suspicion, and accusations coming from both sides in an "us vs. them" relationship, then how does one dismantle "the tree of knowledge of good and evil" in the face of one's enemies?

Confession

"Holy Spirit, I confess that I have had a hateful, unkind, suspicious, resentful, angry attitude towards Moslem people. I choose now with your guidance, help, example, truth, and care to go deeper in getting rid of my hypocrisy, spiritual pride, hatred, and "us vs. them" mentality when it comes to my relationship with Moslem people. They are not the problem; my sins are. I confess these heart maladies and fears rooted in suspicions as wrong, and I ask for your forgiveness and healing. And based on 1 John 1:9 I claim the promise of forgiveness and healing you offer for my guilt and sin. Thank you, Jesus."

Prayer

"Holy Spirit, I give up with your help in faith my judgment, anger, and fear towards Moslem people. I admit that my "us vs. them" mentality is a foundational building block to my unfriendly attitudes towards them. I give this up now in faith, with your help Lord Jesus. I choose to renew my mind with the following humbling truths:

1. A Christian is a sinner with faith.

2. A Christian is a lover who sins.

3. A Christian is imperfect.

4. A Christian is just as susceptible to the seduction of power, war, sex, manipulation, money, and oil as anyone else.

5. Christians have caused just as many wars and injustices as any other religion or culture group in history.

6. A Christian has as many misguided loyalties as anyone else.

Where there is hatred I will plant love; where there is suspicion I will choose to see and believe the best in humanity, and care for all Moslem people everywhere. Thank you, Holy Spirit, for bringing your love into my life. In Jesus' name. Amen.

Going Deeper

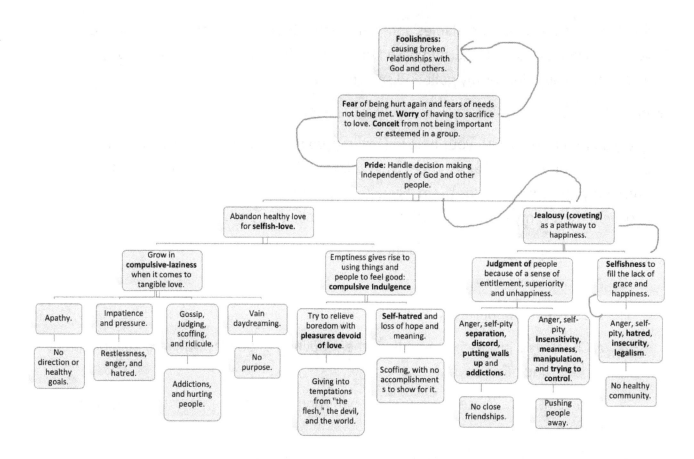

The Sin-Conduit Structure above: "Foolishness=> Fear, Worry, and Conceit=> Pride=> Coveting and Jealousy=> Selfishness=> Hatred" in my life has the following Sin-Anatomy Table:

Hatred	Selfishness	Coveting & Jealousy	Pride	Fear, Worry, & Conceit	Foolishness
	<=	<=	<=	<=	<= Cause and Effect
I'm in the habit of despising, dehumanizing, and demonizing people who have different faith traditions than I do, especially the Moslem people.	Am possessively loyal to a Fundamentalist caricature of Christianity and Jesus as well when it comes to Islam vs. Christianity. Willing to meanly wage a verbal war or assault to convert Moslem sinners to Christianity.	I want Christianity that I'm sold out devotedly loyal to, to be first in every department that is humanly esteemed in the spiritual realm even if it means hurting people.	I know better, see better, and am better than anyone else when it comes to judging the motives of Moslem people.	I fear that Moslem people are out to cheat, lie, and manipulate the world to convert it to Islam.	Islam is black & therefore so are its adherents. Moslem people can't be trusted. I believe the lie that I must not practice the Golden Rule when it comes to Moslem people, because they only take advantage of it.
I am devoid of love for people when I think this way…					
Confession & Repenting in Faith =>	=>	=>	=>	=>	

This leads to processing it with Jesus' help:

Confession and Prayer

"Lord Jesus, I confess that my attitude towards Moslem people is sinful, and I regret hating them, despising, dehumanizing, and demonizing them. Please forgive me. I give this up now in faith, with your help Lord Jesus.

My selfishness and jealousy puts unhealthy fuel on the rivalry between our two spiritual traditions. I'm sorry for my unhealthy part in this and ask for your forgiveness and healing within me. Lord God, I give up this selfishness with your help through faith in you. Thank you.

My blind, arrogant malice knew no bounds when it came to my spiritual pride in this context. Lord God, I give up these unreasonable and pathetic fears with your help. May your will be done on earth as it is in Heaven. I confess, whatever the state of Islam, many Moslem people are humble and peace loving. Lord, I give up maliciously judging Moslem people. I choose to love each Moslem person I meet with warmth, kindness, and caring instead of being suspicious of them and disbelieving their sincerity, kindness, and intent towards me. Please forgive me these sins, Lord God. I'm a sinner. Praying this way has removed the darkness from within me. Thank you Holy Trinity. Amen."

Prayer

"Dear Heavenly Father, I confess that when my peers rejected me in grade school, my pride, identity, and dignity were under attack; therefore my conceit grew and surged within me in an attempt to save my identity. What I wrongly thought was that I was a good person— second to none, especially when it came to those who rejected me. The hurt of rejection motivated vows on my part to not trust anyone and to see the world in an "us vs. them" mentality that atrophied my love, grew my pride, and laid a foundation of fear.

I choose to see my peers from back then with love, tolerance, care, dignity, and peace instead of as enemies worthy of a war cry. I do this with your help Holy Spirit. They are who they are. I forgive them for their part, I forgive myself, and I withdraw my judgment and attack against you Lord God, in this matter too.

Lord Jesus, in faith and with your help, I give up my fears: of being vulnerable, of losing meaning, of being rejected again, and of being hurt all over again. I choose courage, light, love, and caring in place of all this negative, dark stagnancy in my life. I put my full trust, life, and hope into your hands Lord God. I choose to hold onto your promises to forgive me and heal me. Thank you, Holy Trinity."

Another Step

When hurts and malice run deep, they trigger things in related areas regularly. I have found that praying thoroughly for what gets triggered and praying that hurts get healed (i.e. forgiving those who hurt me, forgiving myself, and giving up judgments and attacks towards God) helps restore me to sanity, and in the process, helps to dismantle "the tree of knowledge of good and evil" within me.

Three Revelations

I realized a few weeks later that there was malice within me. I realized that I was not geared to return good for evil —but evil for evil. In fact, I was geared to be mean, angry, petty, anal, and hateful towards those who threatened my security and my happiness. I confessed this sin to God, received His forgiveness intellectually and emotionally, and took hold of my healing through repenting in faith from this unhealthy way of relating to others. I celebrated Jesus' grace and truth instead.

Then I felt a river of tears within me for the hurts others had inflicted on me. And I decided to forgive them because this had never been processed healthily. I found that in thanking God for this healing and for forgiving me I became more connected, joyful, and at peace within. I was very thankful to Jesus.

I also learned that shoving away any malice, bad energy, or judgmental attitudes into the recesses of my heart, thinking it is dealt with, leads to a carnal kind of energy and attitude that masquerades as an insensitive smile on my face. Confessing my exact malice to God, giving up my exact malice and the sin mechanism within, and asking God to displace it, in faith with Jesus' help in prayer, was the wise thing to do. We might have to do this regularly until a trigger, habit or rut is done away with and our minds and hearts are renewed.

Lastly, I became convinced that my unwanted smile was also rooted in the rationalism I adhered to in my poisoned mind, which began with the devil's lies and grew into "the tree of knowledge of good and evil" within me. This rationalism asserts independence from God's wisdom and seeks to supplant and nullify all of God's love, peace, patience, faith, goodwill and hope that is found in Jesus. This rationalism sought to usurp God's place in my heart.

So, what were the antidotes? They were journaling (that lead to deeper fellowship), learning, confession, repentance in prayer, renewing my mind (with God's thoughts) through Scripture, Christian community, the anointing of the Holy Spirit, remaining humble and teachable when it came to my relationships, and bowing to God's input.

Prayer

"Dear Jesus, I confess that I have bought into a rationalism devoid of your perspectives on reality when it comes to my relationships (i.e. the foundation of supernatural love). Because of this I incorrectly judge people, maliciously, arrogantly, proudly, fearfully, and in a wounded fashion every day. I choose through faith in you Lord Jesus, to give up my dependence on rationalism because it does not lead to love, peace, and joy. Out of my rationalism I have scoffed and hated others throughout my lifetime.

I now choose to be dependent on your wisdom, life, love, shepherding, presence, promises, truth, and grace that raises my mind, and heart to where you designed them to properly function.

Thank you for never giving up on me dear God. I embrace you in my heart, and I reject the devil's lies that I know better, more, or what is right, than any other person, or you the Living God, about the wrongs committed against me. I believe in your lordship Jesus.

Please help me to untangle this horrible mess in my heart, my mind, my relating style, my agendas, and my motives so that I can be fully released into freedom as you promised me so long ago. Thank you, Jesus, Father God, and Holy Spirit. Amen."

More Prayer

"Lord God, I confess that I have a weak, self-pitying, lack of confidence and uncertainty. I have such a lack of faith and cowardice when I want to claim what is mine. I also have within me dark energy: a meanness, malice, "eye-for-an-eye" thinking; a polarizing thinking (I'm good vs. their bad) ready to seize what is mine.

At the same time, I want to be a good person, and I feel I should give up what I'm entitled to so I won't be selfish. On the other hand, I want to come down with a machine-like, Terminator force visiting vengeance on people with a "they deserve my wrath" attitude, so I can get what I think I deserve.

I either wimp out saying I should not be so mean and selfish, or I abrasively make waves to get my way while trying to suppress as much of the darkness within me as possible. Lord God, I know I'm believing many things at the same time that are opposing each other here. I don't know how to sort it out all by myself.

Lord God, I confess my darkness and ask for your wisdom and your thoughts, because I'm caught up in a mess that needs cleaning from the inside out. Thank you.

What God Spoke to Me

"Rene, I feel for your situation, and I want to help you straighten out your bent thinking. You are right that being kind is better than meanly demanding your way. You have had a lack of faith that others will respect you and your rights, and you feel justified in fighting for your rights—but in a badly energized way. But if you believe in yourself and in the goodness I have put in all people, appeal to their desire to do what is right and good in a respectful healthy way, then you will be free in this area."

Repenting and Renewing My Mind

"Lord God, I forgive myself for not believing in myself; for believing the lies from the devil that I am a second-rate loser, inept, and always on the losing side. I confess to believing the lies of the devil, and through faith in you Jesus, I give up believing them now. I change my mind and heart with your grace and truth, Lord Jesus. I am now strong and confident I have rights, and I won't wimp out and give them up because my former strategy was ugly. I now have a healthy outlook on myself and others, with a healthy strategy to ask for things. I have rights like all people. And I now have a healthy peaceful place from which to deal with this weak area. The former dark mess inside of me is vanquished. Thank you for healing me,

Lord Jesus. Amen.

A Breakthrough for the Stronghold: Foolishness, Fear, Pride, Jealousy and Judging

As I experienced what was my horrible, ingrained, negative, emotional attitude again for the thousandth time—that manifested itself in my insensitive smile—I finally understood its meaning after decades of mystery. The thought that was triggered in a certain relationship and perfectly matched my feelings said in my consciousness, "What? Am I the donkey, and you the fucking master, god? Fuck, I'm better than you. Screw you!" It was very harsh, judgmental, envious, and proud. And it had its genesis from hurts I reacted badly to from my childhood. I prayed it through as outlined below:

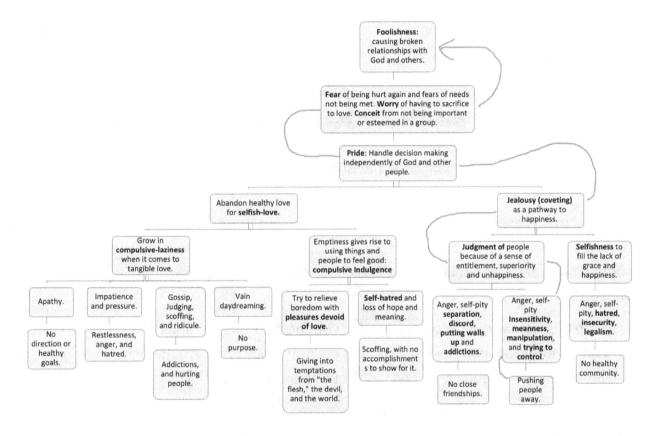

Lord Jesus, I confess my inner Sin-Conduit Structure as being active in many of my relationships: fear, conceit and self-pity leading to pride, jealousy, judging and meanness. I give up self-righteously saying no to them. With your help Lord Jesus, I give up meanly judging people by thinking, "I'm better" and "they're worse" or in believing the lie: "What? Am I the donkey, and you the fucking master, god? Fuck, I'm better than you. Screw you!" With your help Lord Jesus, I give up my scorn which says, "They always think they can order me around by being so disrespectful and conceited." With your help Lord Jesus, I also give up my pride which says, "I'm better than they think I am," which wrongly insinuates they are judging me and helps put me into a box. I give up my fear, self-pity, and conceit. And I take back my identity from the devil; I'm a child of God and made in God's image, with His Spirit within me. Thank you, God.

Lord Jesus, I also admit to the hurt I inflicted to my own identity when I chose to lazily fail the second grade in school because of my sloth, and punished myself for being rejected by my peers in grade school. I forgive myself with your help Lord Jesus, and I receive your forgiveness and healing in this area of my life both intellectually and emotionally. Thank you, Jesus. Amen."

I realized that I needed to renew my mind and attitudes from one of rejecting servanthood to embracing it; I must love others so that I have something to give to those in need—to imitate Jesus' own example in my own small way. Saturating myself in the Scriptures in a teachable fashion was key to renewing my mind as I tapped into what God was specifically speaking to me.

Praying Even Deeper

"Lord God, I confess that I still smile insensitively and judge people. I've said no to it in an attempt to stop, but it does not work so I give it up with your help through faith. Instead I give up the insensitive smiling and judging I do, with your help in faith Jesus. I'm sorry for judging and wanting to condemn people to experience what I went through. I give this up with your help through faith Lord Jesus.

I confess that I have jealousy that says, "I wish I was like normal people who don't have hurts." But this is a lie because everyone has some sort of hurt; this is the truth, and something I need to hear, because it was one more reason why I had trouble empathizing with others.

I give up this jealousy and coveting lie, with your help Lord Jesus, and I choose to love and be kind to others no matter what. I confess my pride that says, "I'm the only one who carries big burdens," and I give it up with your help Lord Jesus.

I admit that I have feared rejection ever since I was first rejected by my peers in South Africa. I give up this fear. And I embrace the truth that I can handle and overcome my negative adversity, with your help Lord Jesus.

My fears spring from the hurt I felt, and I choose here and now to give up my judgments against my South African peers. I forgive myself for lying and causing the rejection in the first place. I also ask for forgiveness for visiting the above lie and the resulting insensitivity on my parents, brother, sister, and others I have met who could have used my comfort and warmth in difficult situations over the years. Thank you for your grace."

Going Even Deeper in Prayer

"Lord Jesus, I confess that I smiled insensitively when I was confronted with an observation from another person today. The thought that matched my smile was, 'What? Am I the donkey and you the pompous ruling elite? I'm better than you." Lord Jesus, please forgive me and heal me; I receive this in faith. Thank you, Lord God. With faith in Jesus, I choose to give up saying no to my judgment, and I instead choose to give up the judgment all through your grace.

Lord God, this means my judgment is growing out of my jealousy of the leadership displayed by the person who broached the observation with me. This jealousy comes from my pride. My judgmental attitude says, "They always think they can set the agenda." And I think way back to Cub Scouts, with me shedding tears because I wasn't chosen for leadership. I thought others should obey me; I wanted leadership and for no other reason. I was hurt because I was rejected as leader (as someone who gets to set the agenda).

Lord Jesus, I give up my judgment on my fellow Cub Scouts from back then, and I give up my childish "beef." I choose to accept their decision to not reward my self-pity, selfishness, and conceit. Lord God, please forgive and heal me from these sins—they are not pretty. I receive your mercy, grace, and healing both emotionally and intellectually. Thank you.

Lord God, I ask you for a tolerant heart, mind, and spirit instead of one that judges people constantly. You are my Savior, because you inspire me with your constant presence, peace, and grace. You fill me with joy, hope, and life. Thank you."

Summary

In all these damaged parts of myself, the Lord showed me that I chose to live life on my own terms, and did as I pleased instead of seeking His will and caring for others. I did this when my peers in South Africa rejected me, and repeatedly thereafter. I had to confess this, give this up, and submit to God. And when I did that, it brought sanity, stability, and peace to my mind and heart.

I'm glad I explored all that grew out of these sins. For the longest time, I had no idea that this one lie was such a huge part of the foundation of "the tree of knowledge of good and evil" within me. I never confessed it to God or repented from it. I always thought it was only my reaction to my peers' rejection of me that was responsible for the mess.

Finally, the Lord led me to own two sins: lying to my peers and trying to use someone to pull it off. I realized these sins were responsible for wreaking havoc on my interior and relational life well into my early 50s. I regretted saying the lie. I confessed these sins to God, I received forgiveness, and I repented from it in faith. Healing came from God and now I thank Jesus that I am at peace. I'm finally free of these wounds and this baggage. There is now closure, and I thank the Holy Trinity. Amen."

11.5: Restoring A Spirit And Attitude Of Worship And Exuberance

After going to a concert, a friend commented that I was like a corpse when it came to expressing appreciation for the music performed. The next Sunday at church I realized I did the same at church during worship. I asked God the question, "Did I make a vow to not celebrate, party, or express appreciation and joy until I'm on the other side of the pearly gate?" He answered, "Yes." This led me to explore the following.

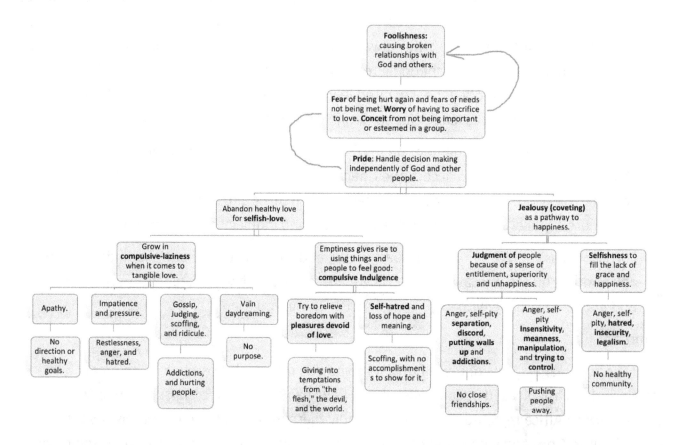

I remember being at church and getting all excited in the worship shortly before my dark night began. But because of the horribleness I experienced with my schizophrenia back then, I did not trust anyone and I became suspicious of my pastor, my church, and the teaching from the Overflowing Grace Conference I had gone to. I decided to withhold any type of celebration from then on until I found relief and security in my mental health like I had known before. I literally gave up living a celebratory life and just started focusing on getting healthy until I prayed the following prayer:

"Lord, I confess that I have held back from celebrating life: giving of myself and taking chances in love; expressing my exuberance, joy, and appreciation; physically worshipping you; and loving others and myself. I have done so because I connected it with getting burned with the schizophrenia. As it got worse I could not stand classical music, nothing had any meaning to me as my mind was taken over by fears and frightening unrealities. I now lay it all before you, and thank you for all the gifts you have given me with this disease, all the people who have helped me as I inched so slowly out of immobility into exercise, out of meaninglessness into involvement and gradually found a way to live, earn a living, be creative, and finally to begin to truly love. I understand now why you took me out of a narrow intellect-focused life of Mathematics, and drew me into a life of faith, understanding and finally love and celebration.

I have done so as a proud and fearful person. Fearful of being hurt and ridiculed and also because of my conceit and cowardice. Lord Jesus, I ask for your forgiveness and healing in this area in my life, and I receive it both intellectually and emotionally. I give up my corpse-like receptivity that has strangled the life, emotions, cares, and joy out of me. Forgive me for holding on to the fear of this aspect of celebration until now. I give up my fears, pride, conceit, and cowardice in this area through faith and with your help, Lord Jesus. Thank you for my friend's observation that finally broke the casket. Help me to live more fully aware of your unconditional love, Lord Jesus."

I also had to confess that I judged both secular and Christian music with bad intentions, both the styles and lyrics together with the listeners. My judging kept me from enjoying a wider variety of music and hindered me from worshipping God more fully. I was sorry and regretted doing so. I then repented in prayer. This brought joy, warmth, healthier energy and more gentleness into my relationships.

11.6: Restoring An Attitude Of Altruism By Going Deeper

The Sin-Conduit Structure below traces out a stronghold against altruism. It goes deeper in dealing with jealousy, and selfishness, along with hatred and the obsessive behavior of attempting to be legalistic in ugly ways amongst other sins:

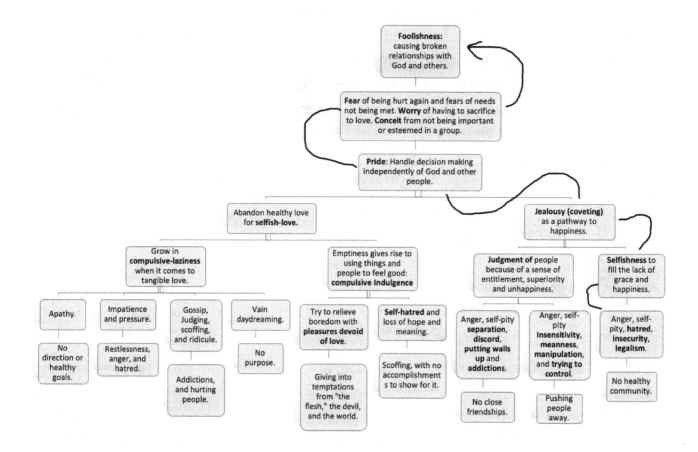

And has the following Sin-Anatomy Table:

Hatred, Self-pity, Angry-pressure	Selfishness	Coveting	Pride	Fear	Foolishness
	<=	<=	<=	<=	<= Cause and Effect
Hate those in my way. Have an "eye for an eye"- mentality against those who frustrate my goals. Plenty of poor-me self-pity. Hard on self and those who take their time seemingly at my expense, and aren't helping my agenda.	Can't live without it. Will do anything to get my way, even when it means being devoid of love. Want things so badly I obsess on them.	I covet so badly stuff that I can't focus on anything else. I'm committed to force, manipulate, and pressure things to get my way.	I am the center of the universe. My ambition comes first; nothing must come in the way of me and my goals.	Motivated by obsessive paranoia, that I might not get what I desire. Don't trust situations and people, afraid of losing the sure thing. I worry and I am anxious when things don't seem to be going my way.	I believe I got to have what my heart is set on no matter what. Nothing can come in the way. Am committed to only focus on my goals and when necessary refuse other people's requests.
Live with black fear, live like a parasite, and am hard on self and others...					
Confession & Repenting in Faith =>	=>	=>	=>	=>	

Prayer

"Lord God, I confess that I hate (or refuse to completely love) those people in the way of my goals. I see those who would hinder me as my enemies worthy of my hostility and revenge. I indulge in plenty of self-pity when things are out of my control. I behave like a parasite. I give these commitments up with your help in faith, Lord Jesus. I am selfishly obsessive to the point of being devoid of love. I covet what I want so badly that I can't focus on anything else except to capture my heart's desires. I regret all of this and give it all up with your help through faith in you, Lord Jesus. I am so proud that my ambition knows no bounds. My happiness comes first. I'm insecure, worry that things won't come through and fearful that I will lose things. Lord God, I regret this all, and I give these attitudes up with your help through faith in Jesus. Lord God, the worst is that I'm "me" centered to the core—"my way or the highway." I'm only focused and committed to my goal—and think "the fuck with everyone else". I regret these commitments and thoughts and give them up now with your help through faith, Lord Jesus. I thank you for forgiving me too. You are God: merciful, kind, and forgiving. Thank you for healing my heart and mind. Amen."

Later on the Lord showed me that I needed to go deeper. He showed me that I often found loving others to be very disagreeable, and that I hated to love in such contexts. I realized that I needed to repent from my attitude of hating to do certain acts of love. Most people like being loved, but not all enjoy loving people. Joy should be a part of loving others. I should love loving people, and when I do I'm embracing and sharing God's grace. When I care for people I will enjoy loving them. If I find doing acts of love hateful, then I will never love in those contexts.

Going Deeper and Conquering More Selfishness

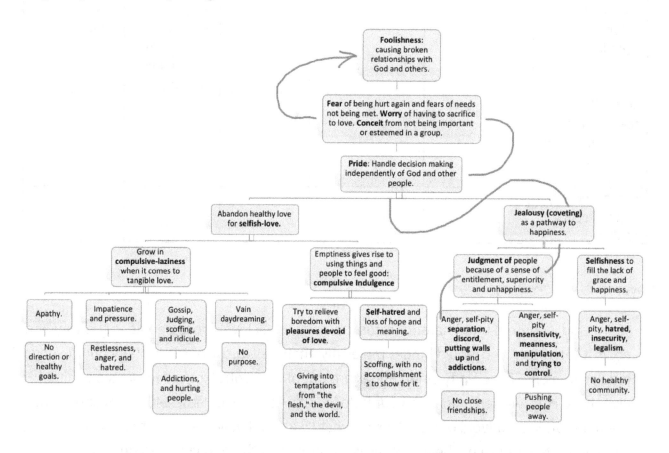

This Sin-conduit Structure has the following Sin-Anatomy Table:

Putting up walls	Judging	Coveting	Pride	Fear	Foolishness
	<=	<=	<=	<=	<= Cause and Effect
Sell off everything and everyone to keep me first or number one in the comfort zone.	Save my life over and beyond that of anyone else's.	Meanly covet a cushy life.	I'm special... must do everything independent of God to preserve my life and comfort.	Fear of being hurt.	Believe the lie that my life means more than any other.
I have treated so many people this way...					
Confession & Repenting in Faith =>	=>	=>	=>	=>	

Praying the Sin-Anatomy Table

Lord God, I give up self-righteously saying "No!" to my selfishness, and instead give it up with your help in this payer. Lord God, I confess that I'm willing to sell everyone else off to save my life. I feel this energy within me. This is very sinful, hateful, evil and malice driven in me — please forgive me Lord Jesus! [Done Rene! Move on!] Thank you Jesus! Lord God I give up this bad attitude with your help and grace through faith in you Jesus!

Lord God, I confess that I have coveted a cushy life — I'm sorry for being so jealously ugly in this attitude. Please forgive me. [Done] Lord God, thanks! Lord God I give up me foolishly and meanly coveting or demanding of a cushy life! I choose to love until it hurts all with your help through faith in you Jesus!

Lord God, I confess that I have plenty of pride connected to this. It says: "I'm most special" and must do whatever to save my life. I confess this is sinful — I regret growing this attitude. Please forgive me Lord God! [Done] Lord God I give it up with your help through faith in you. Thanks!

Lord God I have chosen this form of pride out of fear. Fear of feeling pain, hurt, emptiness and having to pay the price to love. Lord God, I give up these fears with faith in you because you are sufficient, kind and gentle. I'm sorry for waiting this long to come to you to heal my fears. Thanks for being love. Please fill me with your love Jesus. Thanks! [Done]

Lord God, I confess that my life and comfort has meant more than everyone else's including you Holy Spirit. Please have mercy on me Lord God as I don't deserve it. I confess this as sinful, selfish, hollow and empty of meaning. Lord God I give up this commitment to self-absorption, my bad attitude, unholy beliefs, and sinful energy with your help through faith and grace in Jesus. Amen! This leads to what God showed me:

Renewing the Mind

When we focus purely on what we want using war (think anger, meanness, force and threats), then we usually don't care about what our enemy/ neighbor wants. We have become selfish. Realizing that we don't have to go to war and that there are more effective ways to bring peace is where it is at. When we realize and embrace this: non-violence as the better pathway to peace then we begin to care about our enemy/ neighbor and their energy will begin to change for the better too if not already. Unselfish peace becomes ours.

We can be tempted to harden our hearts when our neighbor/ enemy wants to go in what looks like the opposite direction to our goal. When we choose to stomach this at least temporarily we begin to find out slowly that we don't have to be selfish because the detour is also on our way to the goal. When we show kindness to our neighbor/ enemy they will recognize it and they will very likely be determined to show us kindness in return and so help us come to our goal too.

Summary

I could give many more personal examples of using the strategy formulated in this book, but the book would be too long to read if I did. I have used this strategy when it comes to childhood memories, unresolved conflicts with family members, friends, and coworkers and issues that get triggered by strangers on buses or at supermarkets. I have gone deeper and deeper finding lost treasures. Things are gradually getting resolved resulting in peace and love growing in me like God promised me a long time ago.

Erasing bad codes in our hearts and mind is one thing, but they need to be replaced with good codes. Confessing out loud the positive truths the NT speaks about us helps steer us into living out our new identity. Where the tongue goes so does the body.

It may seem that I have been focusing a lot on the Tree Diagrams, but in real life it only becomes the focus when I have been triggered and in need of processing my sin stronghold. In between repenting from one stronghold to another there is a lot of joy, freedom, and celebrating love... yet even in the repentance process there is thanksgiving for mercy and the blessed calm of receiving His grace.

12 Enter The Tree Of Life

There were two trees in the garden of Eden, as recorded in the first book of the Bible[44]. We have looked at one of them in depth—"the tree of knowledge of good and evil." Now we will look at the "Tree of Life".

The "Tree of Life" is not man-made, nor is it fabricated by angelic hands. The "Tree of Life" is Jesus. Jesus is the only foundation that can sustain healthy life, and if we reject Him, we reject life. I have spoken a lot about little "t" truths and how important they are, but without Jesus they become empty philosophies—devoid of power to heal us, make us strong, and give us freedom and peace.

The "Tree of Life" bears good fruit such as love, patience, joy, peace, kindness, goodness, faithfulness, gentleness, and self-control—through the Holy Spirit. We can belong and abide in the "Tree of Life" out of a humble, teachable faith in Jesus. Jesus is the foundation and the structure of the "Tree of Life" as we are one with Him through faith.

"The tree of knowledge of good and evil" is a structure made from commitments to beliefs and expectations based on lies, guilt, fears, anger, and self-pity. It is rooted in wounds from broken relationship that negatively impact our lives, with the building blocks of pride, coveting, jealousy, selfishness, judging, selfish-love, compulsive-laziness, and compulsive-indulging.

The structure that gives life, is rooted in unconditional love that grows with wisdom and truth. It is compassionate, and is based on healthy beliefs, positive commitments, and unselfish expectations that bear good fruit and healthy relationships.

Jesus came that we might have life to the full, and He offers both truth and grace to make it possible. He came to show us that a loving relationship with God, through faith in Him, is the path for that life. Jesus died on a cross once and for all, to save and heal the whole of God's creation. He did not come to condemn, but He came to restore in each of us health, holiness, justice, peace, love, and hope through faith in Him.

The first beatitude found in the Sermon on the Mount that Jesus taught is, "Blessed are the poor in spirit, for theirs is the kingdom of heaven."[45] In today's language this means, "Blessed are the humble, for theirs is the kingdom of heaven." That is what the Sermon on the Mount hinges on. That is what this book hinges on. Not a false humility, but one that is nurtured: through relationship with God, through Jesus Christ, and through faith and grace. "Faith is not a force

---

[44] Cf. Genesis 2:9
[45] Matthew 5:3

that we muster and exert or a technique that gets God's attention and makes Him love us more. No! Faith is like opening a door that lets Jesus into our lives, so we can talk with him and He with us, so that we can have community, and touch one another in love and grow in fellowship."[46] This allows Jesus to guide us into His ways, His feelings, His thoughts, that we might grow in love and be a blessing to others we know now and who we have yet to meet.

Jesus said that if one builds on the Rock (through a living faith relationship with Jesus Himself; with His guidance, empowering presence and grace; and teachings found in The Sermon on the Mount), then one would weather any storm that threatens. Jesus is the blue print for life, understanding, and wisdom. We ought to build our attitudes through a prayerful relationship with Jesus that inspires positive energy, bears healthy actions, and supports life.

The parable of the Mustard Seed[47] is about a seed that is so tenacious that it grows into a tree in the most difficult places (stony hearts), and when it is mature it is able to support the birds of the air. The birds symbolize freedom, life, and people delicately dependent on plenty of patience because life is so often messy, difficult, and fragile. This tree of wisdom and understanding in us is able to support all of this to the glory of God, because it is sustained by God who is ever present. We need to be watered, pruned and cared for so we will grow healthily. The Vinedresser (God the Father) cares for the True Vine (Jesus) and us the branches that choose to remain in Him.

Connection, relationship, and fellowship with Jesus through faith, love, and hope is where life is at, because He promises to never leave me nor forsake me. If all we are focused on are principles, theology, rules, and laws we will miss the grace and peace Jesus wants to pour into our lives. What or who we care about is most important. Learning to distinguish Jesus' voice from others, and to commit to caring for people with His light and guidance is critical. If we reject Jesus, then we don't have life.

The best place to act from is peace. If we don't have it, then we will search for it and sometimes search for it in the wrong places, which can result in idol worship. When we act from the place of Jesus' peace, then we have grace amply supplied, and God does His will through us.

Peace is one of the many fruits of the Spirit we bear. But what about joy? It is wise to be serious about dismantling "the tree of knowledge of good and evil" within and to replace it with virtues and with Jesus' help. *But seriousness taken too far spoils love.*

Another fruit of the Spirit is joy. To attain joy we have to surrender our fears and guilt—both reasonable and unreasonable. When a religious organization requires rashness, inspires

---

[46] Summing up Derek Flood's thoughts in his unpublished book *Intimacy With God*, Cf. pp. 12-13, used with permission.
[47] Cf. Mark 4:31

unhealthy fear, or is too rigid, then there is a good chance we ought to disregard their expectations and move on. We are under grace not law. When joy is finally ours we will be positive, uplifting, confident, and gracious: we will relax and no longer be overly serious about life, relationships, and family; we will choose to play, joke and monkey around; and we will celebrate the simple everyday kindnesses and pleasures that are visited upon people. Joy helps keep the annoying, squeaky wheel oiled. Joy makes us pleasant to be around; it isn't petty, anal, or judgmental because "the joy of the Lord is our strength."[48]

I have spoken much about the "flesh" (sin nature) and the strongholds of sin ("the tree of knowledge of good and evil"), but very little about the devil and the world (system) that both seek to corrupt us. The devil and the world's systems both have voices that try to replace Jesus' voice, direction, care, love, and peace in our lives, with counterfeits and lies. But Jesus gives us a choice in the matter asking us, "Do you want life or death?" It matters how we direct our hunger and thirst, what we enjoy and entertain ourselves with, and why we do the things we do. The choice is ours to make. God's love is unconditional but we will be able to receive according to the choice we make each day.

In an earlier chapter, I mentioned that both the OT and the NT say, "God opposes the proud and gives His grace to the humble." But what does it mean for God to oppose the proud? I think this means that God allows the intrinsic consequences of a proud person's sin to be visited upon the proud person. Sin always goes against love and pushes God away. When we are proud and we get in touch with these consequences from our sins, the consequences are used by God to help convince us of sin's wrongfulness, emptiness, and burdensome costs. One consequence is that we get in touch with our thirst for life, and this can draw us —sometimes pushing, kicking, and screaming all the way—to God, with the help of Jesus Christ. Those who are slowly convinced by God about the consequences of their pride and other sins start to search for real peace, love, joy, and grace in more honest, healthy ways and places.

We see this in Scripture. In the parable of the prodigal child (Cf. Luke 15:11-32), that Jesus shared in His teachings, the father (God) in the parable does not show his youngest child asking for his inheritance any of the following: anger, bitterness, self-pity, meanness, desire for vengeance, or controlling discipline. The father does not threaten, coerce, manipulate, or throw a guilt-trip at his child to get him to stay and tow the family line. Instead he gives his child the opportunity and ability to experience the world, so he will hopefully get to see the consequences of his misguided loyalties, beliefs, decisions, actions and sins.

Abandoning spiritual holiness (sin) creates distance between us and God just like it does between the prodigal child and his father. It's this distance that turns out to be very unpleasant

---

48 Nehemiah 8:10

for the prodigal child, as he gets more in touch with his difficult situation. The father visits the intrinsic consequences of his child's sin on his child by allowing the child to hit rock bottom—to experience both the good and the bad in the world. When a child does hit rock bottom, they remember their father's house, and they begin to long for what they once had. And it is this burden and vacuum that motivates them to search for and make their way back to their father's house in a more humble fashion.

13 Conclusion

Any process to wholeness is a journey, and not a pit stop. I often ask Jesus what He wants me to do next and He often tells me to hope. I finally understand that He means for me to journey with Him, talk with Him through journaling, as things, situations, and people come into my life and help to trigger stuff inside of me. Then as I must deal with issues that come up in my daily life, I may use them as opportunities to further dismantle "the tree of knowledge of good and evil" and reap the resulting spiritual growth. I count this process as pure joy. This is done more healthily by entering into Jesus' peace, believing in and counting on His grace, and standing on His truth.

There are always new things to learn and to grow in the practice of doing; with hope, faith, and love, influenced by Jesus, being the focus.

I am realizing, more and more, that healing comes into my life through forgiving the agents of my hurts one at a time, and by receiving the forgiveness of my sins from God. I also need to jettison fear, conceit, angry pressure and self-pity to dismantle the rest of "the tree of knowledge of good and evil" within me, with Jesus' grace and truth.

None of us are perfect. Those interested in freedom will usually have a number of issues they are aware of that need healing (I've had hundreds). Working on the ones that Jesus points out is key to not getting negative, overwhelmed, or discouraged. We need to always look back and see the work God has done in our lives when our faiths are challenged—and not give up.

Ultimately, Jesus saves us from our sins, and grants His grace so we can love. It is as simple as asking for His grace in faith and believing Him for it that lifts us up into supernatural love. When we fall from this grace, we make the necessary adjustments as spoken about in this book, and ask for His grace to love again, trusting again and living it out again freely. This is all done by becoming dependent on the Christian Scriptures which have a lot more power than this book.

I believe the list of sins mentioned below can be tackled using some of the methodologies and theologies from the contents of this book, by applying them to the "tree of knowledge of good and evil" diagram, and asking God for awareness about the connections, so that confession and strategic prayer can be lifted up to bring healing. Obviously, my strategies in this book have their limitations. Other sources of wisdom, truth, principles, and methodologies from the Christian community will be required for a more thorough interior house cleaning that Jesus requests from us in the Gospels.

I don't intend any judgment, hatred, malice, or meanness towards those who struggle with any of the sins mentioned below; I think we all struggle with some of them in some ways. [49] "Judge not lest I be judged" is my motto. Sin is defined as something that is unhealthy, and no judgments are intended by me in listing some of them here. I am a sinner, and no better than anyone else.

These are sins that can be addressed: lying, cheating, stealing, murder, brutality, brawling, idol-worship, materialism, devaluing people, abusive authority, manipulation, self-righteousness, withholding help from the poor, not helping the weak and disadvantaged, suppressing justice, hypocrisy, verbal abuse, violence, child abuse, rape, pedophilia, witchcraft, malice, hating men, misogyny, disrespecting people, bigotry, and all the different kinds of sexual immorality[50] mentioned in the NT scriptures.

This is where my journey has taken me on so far; where the Holy Spirit has landed me. Things are not stagnant.

One can have many victories and then slip into a sin (and not know immediately why) that one previously had victory over. And also all of a sudden find oneself lukewarm when it comes to the following three important practices found in the Scriptures:

1. I can do all [loving] things through Christ Jesus who strengthens me.
2. Do unto others as I want done to myself [in the context of grace].
3. Going the extra mile.

Finding them more difficult than usual, lacking enthusiasm for them and feeling dry inside!

Confessing, repenting, renewing the mind and growing dependent on Jesus in faith, hope, and love are what is required. So much is connected. One sin can trigger a host of other seemingly unrelated sins, even those we had victory over through the grace of God for some time. So

---

[49] Having broken one command, we have broken the whole Law cf. James 2:10

[50] Sexuality is developmental. Homosexuality is not an outright choice and it isn't genetic either. As far as same sex attraction is concerned there are at least four contexts to focus on to finding healthy sexuality: (1) If one does not feel masculine or feminine enough and are seeking to become more masculine or feminine respectively by pursuing same sex relationships, then praying with this in mind is a key to helping bring healing, (2) If one was sexually abused, then focusing on giving up judgments and hatred towards the pedophile(s) who abused you is the place to start. We often take on characteristics of those we hate, (3) Jumping to identity-labels such as: "gay, homosexual, or lesbian" because one feels a draw to a person of the same sex is unwise. So long as such labels are agreed with they are obstacles to healthy sexual identity, (4) Believing the lie that men know better how to love men sexually than women do; or believing the lie that women know better than men on how to love women sexually can confuse a person's sexual identity (in some people this attraction is weak and with others it is strong). Such lies can make one believe more sexual pleasure is on its way. It is such lies that help cause same sex attraction. Truth is needed to tackle such areas of broken sexual identity. The tools developed in this book lend themselves to dealing with topics like these. It is always important to go deeper where possible.

confessing obvious sins like "lying to others" or "cheating others", and repenting from them in a very short time is advisable because they can be triggers.

A fitting way to solidify victory is to each day spend time with God in prayer, Scripture and worship, telling Him that He is absolutely good, and thanking Him for forgiving us after we have confessed our sins (short lists are advisable) to Him. Becoming teachable by Jesus is the healthy path to take as we spend time with Him consistently all the rest of our days. Learning two-way prayer is so important in making this process work well.

Thanks for taking an interest in what I have written in this book. And thanks for putting up with my constant repetition and emphasis for the need to confess, repent, and renew ourselves interiorly through the grace and truth found in Jesus: with prayer, with the backdrop of scripture, and with the strategies found in this book. I leave you with what I wish for myself and for you all:

> "The Lord bless you
> and keep you;
> the Lord make his face shine on you
> and be gracious to you;
> the Lord turn his face toward you
> and give you peace."[51]

I entrust you to the Lord, and those who will guide you more deeply in the ways of truth, humility, grace and love—and not with empty philosophies. Journaling and using the framework and strategies found in this book are keys that will help one go deeper, repent, and find healing. I encourage you to grow in two-way conversation with God through journaling; to seek God for friendship sake, with the aim of loving people more than concepts.

---

[51] Number 6:24-26

14 Further Reading

I am aware that the approach formed in this book may help some people, but I am sure that it won't help everyone to become completely free and enjoy life the way Jesus intends them to. Here is a list of books I'd recommend that touch on topics I missed or glossed:

(1)   *Can You Hear Me?* by Brad Jersak (ideal for building two-way prayer).

(2)   *Battle Field of the Mind* by Joyce Meyer (ideal for learning to think healthily and positively, and to maintain it).

(3)   *4 Keys to Hearing God's Voice* by Mark and Patti Virkler (ideal for building two-way prayer).

(4)   *Imagine Heaven* by John Burke (ideal for seeing God as love and non-judgmental, and it also gives glimpses of Heaven and Hell).

(5)   *Living Beyond Your Feelings* by Joyce Meyer.

(6)   *The Root of Rejection* by Joyce Meyer.

(7)   *Change Your Words Change Your Life* by Joyce Meyer.

(8)   *Emotionally Free* by Dr. Grant Mullen.

(9)   *Waking the Slumbering Spirit* by John and Paula Sandford.

(10) *Tired of Trying To Measuring Up* by Jeff VanVonderen.

(11) *Soul Repair* by Jeff VanVonderen and Dale & Juanita Ryan.

(12) *Healing the Past Releasing the Future* by Frank & Catherine Fabiano.

(13) *Unbound* by Neal Lozano.

(14) *The Pressure's Off* by Dr. Larry Crabb.

(15) *Freedom from Addiction* by Neil T. Anderson.

(16) *Breaking the Bondage Of Legalism* by Neil T. Anderson.

(17) *Winning the Battle Within* by Neil T. Anderson.

(18) *The Bondage Breaker* by Neil T. Anderson.

(19) *Freedom from Fear* by Neil T. Anderson.

(20) *Liberating Prayer* by Neil T. Anderson.

(21) *Finding God's Will* by Neil T. Anderson.

(22) *When the Spirit Comes in Power* by Peter Herbeck.

(23) *The Twelve Steps: A Spiritual Journey, A Working Guide For Healing*, by Kathleen S.

(24) *Anger: Handling a Powerful Emotion in a Healthy Way* by Gary Chapman.

(25) *Boundaries* by Dr. Henry Cloud & Dr. John Townsend.

(26) *Healing the Wounded Spirit* by John & Paula Sandford.

(27) *Becoming a Family that Heals* by Drs. Beverly and Tom Rodgers,

(28) *Inside Out* by Dr. Larry Crabb,

(29) *Finding God* by Dr. Larry Crabb

ABOUT THE AUTHOR

I lived my early life in South Africa but have lived since then in Canada. I have struggled with schizophrenia since 1992. I have struggled with many addictions. I am still fighting the fight of faith to love people more deeply. If you wish to contact me, then visit: www.brokenintofreedom.ca

BOOKS BY THE AUTHOR

Exploring Faith, Hope & Love
Dismantling the Tree of Knowledge of Good and Evil Within So Love Can Thrive
Contrasting Humility and Pride
Going Deeper With the Twelve Steps
To Be Broken into Freedom: A Spiritual Journey

If you like any of these books please visit an Amazon website to leave a Review.

CPSIA information can be obtained
at www.ICGtesting.com
Printed in the USA
BVHW010919120322
631183BV00014B/28